Is "Modern" Medicine Killing You?

by Dr. Marcus Laux

" In its March 6, 1995 issue, *Time Magazine* reports in an article titled "How to Live to Be 120," the "surprising vigor" of America's senior seniors—85 and older. Says the article: "Between 1960 and 1990, while the overall U.S. population grew 39%, the ranks of those 85 and older jumped 232%."

Some experts project that by the year 2040 there will be 4 million Americans 100 years or older.

Why the upsurge? *Time* quotes Richard Suzman of the National Institute of Aging: "People who live past 85 are a hardy group."

In the same article, Harvard geriatrician, Dr. Thomas Perls asserts that 100-year-olds, "handle stress very well."

Two factors are key, according to the article: Genetics and lifestyle. Your genetic makeup is supported by lifestyle choices that boost your immunity to many stress and age-related diseases. This increases your chances of living a healthy, active life to the end of your genetically predetermined lifespan of 110 to 120 years. **"**

What you should know about Dr. Marcus Laux:

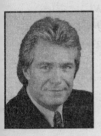

If you were to sit across a coffee table and talk with Marcus Laux, you'd come away feeling that this man is not merely an enlightened physician, but a doctor of uncommon compassion and understanding. The kind of doctor that once moved one patient to write, "God was truly smiling on me that day we met. My life has changed in epic proportions ever since." And still another to confide: "Your faith and help strengthened me, buffered me, inspired me and helped heal me . . . I honor you."

A doctor who believes <u>you</u> are the healer, not him

Marcus Laux is an uncommon practitioner in many ways. He is passionate in his conviction that even though he may be trained as a physician, you are the real healer. You, not he, will improve your health and extend your life. He may be the enlightener, but it is you whose self-healing powers will serve you better than any medical person ever will.

Dr. Laux's understanding of how your body and mind collaborate in this process makes him an invaluable guide to a life of healthy longevity.

An early desire to be a different kind of doctor

During his pre-med undergraduate years at the University of Vermont, Marcus sensed all was not right with the medical profession. There were a few doctors he truly admired, but many more he felt were there just for the high earning potential. They seemed to have no real connection with their patients, viewing them primarily as separate body parts to be treated rather than as whole human beings. As he puts it, "The nurses were the only ones who really gave compassionate care to patients. The doctors were engaged in treating symptoms, writing endless prescriptions, checking their investment portfolios and bragging about their golf games...I didn't fit in."

A discovery that changed everything

It wasn't until some years later that Dr. Laux discovered natural or *naturopathic* medicine, based on a combination of modern medicine and natural healing philosophies. It was a discipline, he found, that emphasized care of the "whole person", recognizing influences such as nutrition, lifestyle habits, emotions and environment on a patient's natural healing ability. The ultimate aim was to help people take more control over these factors to influence their health and longevity. This future doctor knew he had found a home.

How to learn from Dr. Laux

After receiving his degree in Naturopathic Medicine, Dr. Laux went into private family practice. He became passionately interested in the field of longevity and combating age-related disease. He speaks at forums across the country, and tens of thousands subscribe to his monthly letter, *Naturally Well*.

For his first book, *Is "Modern" Medicine Killing You?*, Dr. Laux has chosen a question-and-answer format, anticipating questions you might have about this exciting and promising area of health and healing.

TABLE OF CONTENTS

CHAPTER 1

Prescribe Your Own Medicine and Live Longer

You have the power to do more for your good health and longevity than anyone else—including your doctor. Why?

Because the diseases we fear most—cancer, heart disease and stroke—are principally diseases of lifestyle. They are brought on by the way we eat, the unhealthfulness of our environment, and often by the stresses in our daily lives. You can neutralize all these factors—with less sacrifice than you might imagine. That's why I wrote this little book. To show you how, with minimal effort, you can bring about changes that extend your life—and good health—longer than you ever imagined possible.

Doctor, nobody I know has lived much beyond 75 or 80. How can I take aim at 120, and stay healthy besides?

You have the good fortune to be alive at the beginning of a new frontier in natural medicine and enlightened immunology. So you may want to reconsider any assumptions you've made about the inevitability of old-age illness, decrepitness and decline.

Reason: They're probably assumptions based on the conventional, outmoded, even primitive reasoning of Orthodox Medicine.

The recent discoveries you will read about in this book will convince you beyond a doubt that you can and should aim for a human being's natural biological life expectancy of 110-120 years.

But what should I know about living longer that my doctor hasn't already discussed with me?

Unfortunately, as well-meaning, dedicated and professional as many doctors are, most have little, if any, formal education in preventive medicine.

Reason: 90% of medical schools don't offer or require the subject. (I'll explain the disturbing reasons why later.) In fact, a conventional doctor's education in prescription drugs and their effects comes mostly from drug company advertising. This is unfortunate to say the least, and potentially dan-

90% of medical schools don't stress preventive medicine

gerous. Especially with drugs that have powerful, toxic side effects.

Scary result: It may
explain why drugs pre-
scribed by doctors and
approved by the FDA
kill 146,000 people each year.

**FDA-approved drugs
kill 146,000
people annually.**

Is this an indictment of the whole medical community?

Not at all. I have dear friends who are conventional doctors, including a number who have
begun recommending naturopathic therapies in
their practices. But I must make a rather shocking statement to a lot of Americans now under
the care of devoted—yet unenlightened—medical professionals:

Warning: There are a lot of you who may be
slowly dying, inch by inch, year by year, through
your relationship with a duly licensed, yet con-
ventionally educated M.D. It's sad, but that's
how clueless and misguided conventional medicine often is about treatment and prevention
(much more on this later). But all is NOT lost.

The good news: As you go through this
book, you will uncover highly-effective *drug-
sparing* and non-surgical alternatives that enable
you to realistically look forward to a much

longer, much healthier life—and to reset your biological clock for an age well into the next century.

Most people feel that living longer usually means surviving in a hospital or nursing home. Your response?

I urge you to reconsider that idea as well, and I'll tell you why: Even though living that kind of life—or "existence" is more like it—has been the norm for many older folks in the past, it needn't be that way any longer.

Reason: Clinical studies have shown that by taking the right steps, prolongation can occur in the vital, active portion of life, while extending the elderly portion relatively little. For you, "old age" can be youthful and beautiful, free of disabling illnesses like heart disease, stroke, arthritis and osteoporosis, to name just a few.

So what's the key to healthy longevity?

It's not having a great doctor. Or a medicine chest full of wonder drugs. It's not always having "good genes", for they

The answer is a marvel of nature

cannot guarantee the quality of a longer life. Instead, it's having the most powerful protector of all: a well-functioning immune system. And in these pages you'll learn simple steps to make sure this marvel of nature is always doing the job you want it to do.

No one can guarantee you healthy longevity—yet. But that guarantee is getting closer, probably in your lifetime. And we've already unlocked many of the doors—now we simply have to walk through them. One guarantee I <u>CAN</u> make: By reading this book, you'll gain information that will substantially *increase* your chances for a long, healthy lifespan.

What benefits can I reasonably expect by taking life-extending measures starting tomorrow?

If you're in your so-called "senior" years, not only can your life span be extended, but so, too, can the quality and energy of your life. So while other seniors you know may prefer siestas over fiestas, it'll definitely be the other way around for you. If you're middle aged, you can regain some of your youth as well as dramatically

You'll prefer fiestas over siestas

improve the quality of your life and stretch your life span. And if you're young, the duration of your youthfulness can extend far into the future.

What's the best first step to take?

I'd say prepare your mind to live longer and live healthier. In other words, "psych" yourself up for this adventure. Because your beliefs will have a tremendous effect on what you're able to do with your life.

Reason: There is abundant biological evidence that positive thoughts rally the body's natural immunity against age-associated disease. I'll share more with you about this phenomenon later in this book.

EASY REMINDERS:

- You can do more for your own good health than any doctor.

- There are highly-effective drug-sparing techniques most doctors don't know about.

- Life extension prolongs the active pleasurable portion of your life, not the time you survive in a nursing home.

- Prepare your mind to live longer, because "psyching" yourself up rallies the body's natural immunities.

CHAPTER 2

A Discovery That Will Have a Major Impact on Your Health

There are miracle substances you're going to hear more and more about in coming years called phytochemicals. The term means "plant chemicals" and, while they've been with us for millions of years, our new understanding of them is the most important development in preventive medicine and nutritional science in years—perhaps even surpassing the discovery of vitamins and antioxidants.

Even though vitamins and antioxidants remain a key part of your defense against disease, phytochemicals will be the aggressive leader of that defense.

What should I know about phytochemicals?

They are a set of compounds found naturally in plant and vegetable life and they pack a disease-preventing wallop. Unfortunately, we've branded them with tongue-twisting labels that are hard for the average person to remember, like Coumarins, Dithiolthiones and Limonene (makes you want to throttle the botanical chemists who name them!). But their power is stunningly simple: They are nature's most powerful immunity enhancers.

What they do: In the wild, phytochemicals protect plants from harmful sunlight, from

A helping connection between species

"bugs" like viruses and bacteria, and from real bugs as well. Some say it is merely a quirk of nature that they also help people. Perhaps. But I'm convinced that it's more evidence of the many helping connections between species... connections that we are only just learning about.

How exactly do they protect humans?

Research has only skimmed the surface, but so far we know that phytochemicals have been shown to "pump up" your immunity against both heart disease and osteoporosis, as well as killers like lung, esophageal and colon cancer. And that's just the prevention side. Amazingly, these substances also perform miracles for those who already have disease.

Proof: According to Devra Lee Davis, senior science advisor at the U.S. Public Health

Service, "There is growing evidence that these natural products can take tumors and defuse them...they can turn off the proliferation process of cancer."

How much can I expect to reduce the risk of cancer by consuming phytochemicals?

I'd say quite a bit. The research has compared the eating habits of people with and without cancer. Those who consumed the most phytochemically-rich foods were about half as likely to have cancer as those who ate the least.

What do plants know that we don't?

Since they've inhabited this planet far longer than us, these plants have had a big head-start in learning how to survive. They are master biochemists producing sophisticated agents for their own protection

Plants are revealing their survival wisdom to us

and healing. And now they are revealing that survival wisdom to us.

What do they do in my body?

Not surprisingly, they work in your system just the way they work in plants, as immunity boosters to safeguard against foreign invaders.

When we consume the plants, they pass along their own miracle protection.

Example: Penicillin is an antibiotic originally manufactured by a plant—the lowly soil fungus—to protect itself from harm.

Now it does the same for us.

What should I eat to get the best phytochemical protection?

Just to pick one food that takes rather aggressive action—Broccoli. It has a phytochemical compound that boosts the production of anti-cancer enzymes within hours of being eaten. So when you swallow something that may have cancer-causing properties (especially as relates to colon cancer),

Carcinogens are detoxified and swept out of your body

the enzymes seek it out immediately and detoxify it before it can harm you. Cabbage and cauliflower give you the very same protection.

Extra advantage: Phytochemicals aren't lost as often through cooking as some vitamins are. In fact, when you cook broccoli you are likely to *enhance* its phytochemical potency! That's because there's a particular enzyme that needs to "leap" from one set of cells to another for maximum effect. Cooking makes that happen.

Extra advantage #2: It doesn't matter if you buy the vegetables fresh, canned, frozen, juiced or peeled. You still get a full measure of phytochemical protection. (Anybody for a glass of broccoli juice?)

[NOTE: There is much more you need to know about phytochemicals than can be covered here, so I have recently published a Special Report, *Naturally Immune for Life* in which I identify the most important phytochemicals discovered thus far, the best plant sources for them and, equally important, what kind of protection each one has shown to provide. Look in the back of this book to see how you can receive a free copy.]

What about "antioxidant" supplements—will I need them now?

I highly recommend antioxidant supplement "insurance," just to make sure you get the protection you may not be getting in your diet. After all, if the nutrition is not in a vegetable's soil, it's not in the vegetable. And because

Antioxidants are extra armor against cancer

many of our fruits and vegetables are grown in demineralized soils and then subjected to pesti-

cides and the "torture" of long storage and pro-
cessing, some may be nutritionally depleted by
the time they reach your table.

Easy vitamin formula: I always say, "take
your ACEs"—vitamins A, C and E—to keep
your immune system's armor against dreaded
cell oxidation (aging) and cancer at its most
resilient.

Most potent: Did you know there's a fruit-
derived substance that has 50 times more antioxidant activity than vitamin E, and 20 times
more than Vitamin C? It's true. It is non-toxic
and is highly effective even after long term use.
What is it? Where can you get it? (Get ready for
another tongue-twister...) It's Oligomeric
Proanthocyanidin and can be found in either Pro-
N-30 from Orange Peel Enterprises (800/643-
1210) or Grape Seed Phytosome from
Enzymatic Therapy (800/783-2286). You can
probably find both of these in your local health
food store.

EASY REMINDERS:

- Phytochemicals from plants have been shown
  to pack a wallop in protecting you from killer
  diseases.

- They've also shown the ability to shrink tumor

growth and stop the spread of cancer.

Broccoli, cabbage and cauliflower have phyto-chemicals that work fast to defuse cancer-causing substances you make take in.

Vitamin supplements are important insurance to make sure you're getting ample protection.

For more information on phytochemicals, request the free Special Report, *Naturally Immune for Life*. See the back of this book for details.

CHAPTER 3

Wash Pesticides and Drug Toxins Right Out of Your Body

They're life-shortening and a drain on your immune system...and they compete with all the immunity-enhancing measures you take. But, unless you buy organic foods, it's still hard to completely escape plant pesticides and drug toxins in your life.

Other bad guys: Antibiotic-engorged beef and poultry wouldn't be necessary if processors could figure out how to make a buck and still raise healthier, cleaner animals. (If you could see their living conditions, you'd lose your appetite.) As for the drug companies, we might have to censure a few CEO's to get some action. In the meantime, there are some things you can do to avoid contamination from additives and toxins.

What's your advice on keeping my body free of the poisons that get into food?

Start, of course, by "going organic" as much as possible. Even though natural organic vegetables and meats are often more expensive, it's worth every extra penny to be relatively free of pesticides, chemicals, steroids and antibiotics. Plus, organic foods can *contain up to 200% more nutrients.*

Organic food is 200% more nutritious

Double trouble: We now know that indiscriminate use of human antibiotics impairs our immunity and breeds killer "bugs" (see more on this in chapter 8). But when you multiply that threat by consuming animals dosed with antibiotics (to keep them from succumbing to their poor living environment), it spells big trouble for your ability to ward off serious disease.

Pesticide alert: Many agricultural pesticides have an estrogenic effect on your body—they mimic estrogen. This added excess is implicated in several types of cancer, weight gain in women and feminization in men (resulting in possible decreased penis size and lower sperm count).

But how do I "de-fang" toxins and pesticides that slip unavoidably into my system?

Since such prevention is key to longevity, I recommend you take *green superfoods,* one of nature's most protective and nutrient-rich food sources. Green superfoods are heavily laden with chlorophyll, which has the ability to neutralize and remove toxic pesticides, drug residues and other unwanted chemicals from your body.

How Effective?: Let me give you an idea of the awesome power of at least one superfood to "de-tox" your system. Spirulina—a special form of blue-green algae—is now being used in the former Soviet Union to reduce radiation poisoning in some 160,000 children who were innocent victims of the Chernobyl nuclear plant disaster.

Results: Based on tests of a sampling of children at the Institute of Radiation Medicine in Minsk, the Russian Ministry of Health concluded that "Spirulina pro-

Chlorophyll is a super scavenger of internal toxins

motes the evacuation of radionucleides from the human body." Doctors found that fully 83% of the kids given Spirulina over 45 days had a marked decrease in the amount of radioactivity in their urine.

Does that mean it can protect ME from radiation, too?

Yes. Besides neutralizing chemical toxins,

these miracle green substances give you extra protection from exposure to atmospheric radiation of all types—from the emissions of power lines to microwave ovens to garage door openers and even computers and TVs.

Unexpected benefit: Because green superfoods are so efficient at detoxifying the body, they can, for example, help arthritis sufferers by relieving the immune system of its pollution-fighting tasks in order to repair joints (See more on this in Chapter 10.)

Do I have choices in green superfoods?

Yes—and they're all quite powerful. You can select from the following: Alfalfa, Barley Grass, Wheat Grass, Blue-Green Algae, Chlorella and Spirulina. Spirulina, incidentally, has 60% complete digestible protein, more than any other food on the planet.

So much for *inner* "pollution"—is there a way to overcome the effects of polluted air?

Good question, because environmental pollutants pervade—and shorten—our lives. However, even though you can't avoid air pollution completely if you live in an urban or suburban area, there are ways to greatly minimize the risk.

Solution: My recommended daily "cocktail" of antioxidant ACE vitamins is an ace pollution and

A vitamin cocktail that beats smog

ozone fighter, fending off the free radical formation you've read about that "rusts" our cells and causes diseases of aging.

These supplements also prevent—and even repair—long term lung and cellular damage.

Are there also pollutants in my home that affect me?

Unfortunately, yes. Most people don't realize it, but your home can be a minefield of chemical pollutants.

Furniture, carpets, insulation, paint and even fireplaces can emit hazardous gases you can't smell, but are responsible for health problems from sore throat to cancer.

Watch out: Formaldehyde, for example, is a carcinogen released from a whole bunch of household items such as particleboard (used to make bookcases, desks and tables), foam insulation, upholstery, curtains and from other unsuspected sources.

Is there a remedy?

You could buy an expensive room air cleaner, but there's an easier, cheaper, more natural solution. Ordinary houseplants such as the Boston Fern, English Ivy and Spider Plants are

Nature's crack pollution-buster is a houseplant

Mother Nature's crack pollution-busters, and do a super job of filtering toxins from your home. This is particularly important during winter months when you are likely to spend most of your time closed up indoors with the windows shut.

Example: A single Boston Fern can remove approximately 1,800 micrograms of formaldehyde from the air per hour (an amount one might find in a typical 10 ft. by 10 ft. room). That's sufficient to completely clean the room of pollutants, according to tests by the Environmental Protection Agency. Put one in your living room, den and in each bedroom for maximum protection. In addition to adding natural beauty to your home, introducing such plants can significantly reduce the concentration of harmful chemicals your body takes in and attempts to detoxify.

EASY REMINDERS:

- Pesticides and toxic drug residues are a drain on and can paralyze your immune system.

- You can't escape them completely if you live in a city or suburb.

- Buy organic products as often as possible to avoid pesticides, growth hormones and antibiotics.

- Green superfoods like Spirulina and Barley Grass "de-fang" toxins that get into your system.

- A daily "cocktail" of Vitamins A, C and E help shield you from environmental toxins.

- Houseplants can detoxify and clear chemical pollutants in your home.

CHAPTER 4

Foods to Avoid to Prevent Premature Aging

It's a little scary, but the aging effect that some foods have on your body has been described as "internal radiation". We know how dangerous high-energy radiation can be, as in the effect on the children of Chernobyl that I spoke of earlier. The immune system is compromised through free-radical formation and victims become far more susceptible to cancer, arteriosclerosis and stroke—all diseases associated with aging. These same diseases and their aging effects can result from some of the foods we eat.

That's the bad news. The good news is that you can limit or completely avoid the effect of internal radiation by avoiding certain foods—and by consuming others.

What should I steer clear of at mealtime if I want to live longer?

Here's the easiest mealtime formula to live by: The more animal you eat, the more aging and disease. The more vegetable you eat, the less aging and the more good health.

Important: This doesn't mean you have to become a vegetarian. It simply means minimize the meat portion of your life and maximize the veggie portion.

Are there any foods I should NEVER eat?

If I had to pick one, it would be margarine. Margarine is absolutely foreign to the human digestive system and compromises your immune system. (Even rodents won't eat it!) But that doesn't mean you can't still "butter" your toast in the morning. See the next chapter for a surprise alternative.

Excess saturated fats shorten your life

I'd also go light on fried foods. They're *really* hard for your body to digest.

Also remember: any substance that contains an excess amount of saturated fat is ultimately a life-shortening substance.

I love a nice juicy hamburger once in a while — how much is that going to age me?

Not much, if at all. I love a good burger myself, but I must tell you the average hamburger is full of free radicals because it contains a high percentage of saturated fat (that's what makes it "juicy"). So what to do for your burger craving? Easy—buy and use fresh lean ground beef.

Extra juicy: If you want your burger especially juicy, brush on a bit of olive oil. Olive oil is a delicious monounsaturated fat not associated with cancer or heart disease.

Can I aim to be a healthy 120 if I sneak saturated fat into my life?

You needn't "sneak." There's really nothing wrong with saturated fat in your diet. It's only a problem in excessive amounts, especially through highly fatty oils added to your foods. The only real sacrifice you need to make is avoiding processed foods containing palm oil, coconut oil and hydrogenated or partially-hydrogenated oils.

Just say no to anything with tropical oils

Reason: They're fats that extend a product's shelf life, but they shorten your life. You'll find them in candy bars, evil margarine, some cookies and non-dairy creamers.

Stay clear of those and you'll be much better off.

I do see the term "hydrogenated or partially-hydrogenated oil" in a lot of processed food. What exactly does it mean?

You may not want to know. It's a process of turning vegetable oil from an organic substance into an inorganic one—from a live to a dead concoction—to keep it from breaking down and becoming rancid while sitting for long periods on a grocer's shelf. In effect, hydrogenation *plasticizes* the oil, allowing it to preserve the shape and consistency of the food it's in. The process also produces trans fatty acids (as in margarine), directly linked to heart disease and high cholesterol.

What do you say to a salt lover who refuses to give it up?

I say, don't. Yes, do avoid ordinary table salt. It deserves the bad rap it's gotten and is linked to all sorts of problems including depression, pre-

menstrual tension, migraines and bloating. Worse, it can usher in kidney disease as well as the

How to avoid the "silent hit-man"

"silent hit-man", high blood pressure. Salt substitutes are not satisfactory to a lot of people.

Instead: use Celtic brand sea salt obtained from evaporation of ocean brine. It has an exquisite flavor and a wealth of minerals.

Little-known secret: It's a product called Bragg Liquid Aminos—but don't let the name confuse you. It is WONDERFUL for adding the salty flavor to foods without the salt. Use it on veggies, rice, beans, soups, wok and stir frys, meats, poultry and fish. Plus it contains 15 healthful amino acids! You can buy it at any health food store.

EASY REMINDERS:

- The aging effect that some foods have on you is like "internal radiation"—but you can avoid it.

- The more animal you eat, the more you age The more vegetable you eat, the less you age.

- NEVER eat margarine. And lighten up on fried foods.

- There's nothing wrong with having a juicy hamburger once in a while, but brush on olive oil for the "juice" if desired.

- Avoid processed foods with the following oils: palm, coconut, hydrogenated or partially-hydrogenated oils.

- Use Celtic sea salt and Bragg Liquid Aminos for healthful "salty" taste.

CHAPTER 5

My Longevity Diet: Butter, Beer, Sloppy Joes and "Twinkies"!

I'm bored by bland food...so when I'm hungry and sit down to a meal I want food that excites my taste buds. On the other hand, food that should be keeping all of us nourished and healthy often is making us sick.

Reason: Our bodies don't know what to do with our diet of "refined" food, fake food and non-food. So it clogs up our system and contributes to all sorts of problems, some ultimately fatal.

Yet when someone suggests "healthful alternatives" it immediately translates as dull and tasteless. What to do?

The answer is to uncover natural food choices that taste as good or better than the stuff that's bad for you.

How can I use butter and not "gunk up" my arteries with fat?

Do what I do: Use a clarified form of butter

called ghee. It's delicious—most agree it's even better. Milk solids have been removed to form clarified butter, and the purified product actually has healing properties. It's available from Purity Farms at many health food stores. [NOTE: See my recipe for "Twinkies" made with ghee at the end of this chapter. Also my recipe for heart-healthy Sloppy Joes.]

Even better: Olive oil is also a truly delicious and healthful butter replacement. Nowadays, it even comes in a spray for more convenience (like putting it on toast in the morning).

What is olive oil's link to longevity?

This is a truly remarkable food. I call it the lubricant of longevity. Many studies have shown that populations using large amounts of olive oil—such as in Italy and Greece—have much lower rates of heart disease and stroke.

Olive oil lowers the "bad" cholesterol

Reason: Olive oil is the richest monounsaturated fat, and has been proven to lower cholesterol, especially LDL, the "bad" cholesterol.

But the benefits of this oil don't stop with your cardiovascular system. There's strong evidence that it retards cancer growth as well, in particular, breast cancer.

Explanation: Olive oil is rich in Vitamin E, one of the best antioxidants for resisting the invasion of cancer-causing free radicals.

It also has other connections to a longer life: Olive oil has shown in studies to slow down the normal wear and tear on vital organs—including the brain.

Fascinating fact: This link between olive oil and longevity is further strengthened by the fact that olive trees have been known to live as long as 3,000 years!

How on earth does beer contribute to a longer life?

Believe it or not, beer can help reduce your overall cholesterol level and thus keep clots from forming in your arteries.

Reason: Moderate amounts of alcohol have been shown in numerous studies to be a pretty adept cholesterol fighter. However, I do prefer you drink such beers as Anchor Steam, Samuel Adams, Sierra Nevada or any Bavarian beer because they are naturally fermented, organic and chemical free, whereas many other brands use formaldehyde to kill the fermentation process. If you prefer wine over beer, red wines appear to have the same cholesterol-lowering properties. If you don't happen to be a wine drinker, you can enjoy plain purple concord grape juice and get the same benefit. It contains the same substance (resveratrol) that red wine offers for lowering serum cholesterol.

What foods do you especially recommend for an anti-aging lifestyle?

The best foods for longevity are what Mother Earth has deliciously prepared for us— WHOLE foods like vegetables, grains (including whole-grain pastas, breads and cereals), beans (and other legumes like lentils), seeds and fruits and nuts.

Reason: Your digestive system is essentially the same as your ancestors had 50,000 years ago. It is designed for the foods provided by your habitat. Today's highly processed foods, with unnatural amounts of fat, sugar, salt and all those unpronounceable food chemicals are still very new to our system.

Your digestive system is 50,000 years old

It's kind of like putting unleaded fuel into a vintage car and expecting it to run efficiently.

But what if you're addicted to the taste and convenience of processed foods?

Nowadays, you can have many of the tastes you truly enjoy, but in foods that nature gave us. Not only do easy-fixin' recipes abound that mimic the flavors you like, but health food supermarkets now offer many, many frozen, microwaveable

You can get healthful fast-food from the store

entrees you can cook in minutes. Even mainstream supermarkets are carving out areas of their freezer sections for these healthful alternatives.

Reason: They're getting the message that more and more people are turning away from processed foods and toward nature's own bounty. Because not only do whole foods pump up your immune system and prevent age-related disease, but specific foods are natural remedies for a whole range of health problems.

[NOTE: I offer readers of this book an additional free Special Report *250 Mouth-Watering Food Remedies for What Ails You* in which I catalog a whole range of tempting foods that have shown to prevent and cure physical problems.]

I can pick out good vegetables, but are there any grains that are especially good for my body?

Personally, I'm a barley lover. In the Middle East, barley is one of the most important food staples, sometimes called "medicine for the heart."

Barley is called "medicine for the heart"

Reason: It is full of beta glucans, a type of fiber that can lower the risk of heart disease by lowering LDL, the "bad" cholesterol. Barley also contains natural chemicals called protease inhibitors that attack potential cancer-causing agents in our bodies.

Shopping tip: always look for the term "pearled" barley on the box. That's the hull-less variety containing the largest amount of beta glucans.

How to prepare barley? The easiest way is to simply boil it, but instead of using water, I cook it in canned broth for a delicious added flavor. Incidentally, I also make a 'mean' mushroom-barley soup that I share with you in one of my free Special Reports.

If beans are "nature's most perfect food," what about the gas problem?

You're right—all is not exactly perfect with the world's most perfect food. But since beans are as close to good medicine as food can get, let me explain how the gas problem is very easily remedied. Start by eating just a small amount at a meal, perhaps a half cup, even mixed with rice. Then, gradually increase your consumption day by day.

Beans are food as good medicine

Reason: This gives the body a chance to adapt and create enzymes which overcome the gas problem. It's that simple. Another way is to boil the beans for ten minutes, drain the water off, then cook according to directions.

How do beans contribute to health and robust immunity?

Let me count the ways: 1. high in protein, 2. high in fiber, 3. high in complex carbohydrates (for increased energy), 4. high in vital nutrients, like potassium, iron and thiamine and 5. very low in fats and sodium.

You recommend onions over any drug, aspirin included, to prevent stroke and heart attack. Why?

A small amount of raw or cooked onion performs as a natural anticoagulant that helps prevent life-threatening blood clots leading to heart attacks or strokes.

Amazing results: In a landmark study by researchers in India, test subjects were purposely fed fat-intensive meals that raised their cholesterol to dangerous levels, increasing the risk of clots. After a scant two ounces of onion was introduced to their diet, cholesterol was quickly brought within safe limits.

Other researchers have shown that as little as half an onion will boost HDL, the "good" cholesterol by a whopping 30%. Says the author of *The Food Pharmacy,* Jean Carper:

A mere 2 oz. of onion lowered cholesterol

"The onion is one of the best-tested miracle foods of the food pharmacy . . ." I couldn't agree more, especially when you consider the possible adverse effects of blood-thinning pharmaceuticals like aspirin.

You've spoken of apples as the immunity snack of the ages. Why?

The old "an apple a day..." rhyme is one you should stick on your refrigerator door, because it's true. Here are some of the potent healing powers of apples:

a. They beat back both LDL-"bad" cholesterol- and high blood pressure (better in women than men, for some reason).

b. The juices in a fresh apple are strong virus fighters.

c. They're natural appetite suppressants, with enough nutritive value to keep you from having to eat anything else for a low-cal meal.

Apples DO keep the doctor away

d. They're brimming with natural acids that have successfully blocked cancer formation in lab tests.

Fact: Some people benefit from apples just from sniffing them. Yale University researchers found in studies that the scent of spiced apples produced a calming effect which helps to lower blood pressure!

EASY REMINDERS:

- Use a clarified form of butter called ghee, it's delicious AND healthy.

- Live longer using olive oil instead of conventional butter.

- Moderate amounts of alcohol in beer and wine help keep your arteries free of clots.

- Whole foods are great for your body, and now they're being made into tasty convenience foods.

- Barley and beans are just two whole foods with a lot of benefits.

- Onions are an especially powerful cholesterol fighter.

- Apples DO keep the doctor away.

- For more information on the foods that are natural remedies, request an additional free Special Report, *250 Mouth-Watering Food Remedies for What Ails You.* See back of this book for ordering.

DR. LAUX'S SLOPPY JOES

Sauté in 2 tablespoons of ghee:
1/2 cup minced onions

1/2 cup chopped green pepper

When these are slightly limp, add:

1-1/2 lbs. extra lean ground beef, turkey or chicken

Cook and stir until meat is lightly browned.

Add:

1/2 cup chopped mushrooms

2 to 4 cups chili sauce

Sea salt to taste, or Bragg Liquid Aminos

Cook, uncovered, over low heat until the mushrooms are done. With this hot mixture, pour over:

4 slightly toasted whole wheat hamburger buns, sliced and open faced.

DR. LAUX'S HEALTHY (AND DELICIOUS) "TWINKIES"

The cake part:

4 eggs, or equiv. egg substitute

1/2 cup honey

1 teaspoon vanilla extract

3/4 cup whole wheat flour

3/4 teaspoon baking powder

1/4 teaspoon salt

The filling part:

1/4 cup ghee

2 tablespoons canola oil

1/4 cup raw honey

1 teaspoon vanilla extract

1/4 cup nonfat dry milk powder

1/4 cup ice water

1 teaspoon lemon juice

Preheat oven to 375 degrees. Oil and flour 10 x 15-inch pan

Beat eggs until very foamy.

Pour in honey and continue to beat.

Add vanilla, flour, baking powder and salt.

Pour smooth batter into pan, bake 12-15 min..

When cool, loosen with spatula and turn onto flat surface.

For filling, beat softened Ghee, oil and honey with a mixer, finally adding vanilla.

In another bowl, beat milk powder and ice water until foamy, then add lemon juice and beat until the consistency of whipped cream.

Add creamed ghee mixture and beat until thick.

Slice cake like a sandwich, fill with cream and cut into "Twinkie" proportions.

CHAPTER 6

Why Most Doctors Don't Have a Clue or, Worse, Keep You in the Dark

It's a sad fact...as I said in the beginning of this book, that many, many people today may be slowly killing themselves through their relationship with their orthodox physician. Why? How? Few physicians today have any formal training in preventive medicine and have only about four hours of nutritional training scattered over four years of medical school.

Confirmation: In 1985, the President of the American Medical Student Association testified: "Medical education has traditionally focused on the principles of acute episodic health-care delivery, overlooking the concepts and applications of nutrition and preventive medicine."

Why is my doctor so under-trained in preventive medicine?

There are a number of possible reasons.

1) *Intern factories:* Medical schools basically

stamp out future interns, because hospitals need them to staff the front line. That's why the emphasis is on "acute episodic" emergency room skills.

2) ***"Soft" specialty:*** Medical schools teach that medicine has two sides—hard and soft. The hard, or critical side, is surgery, prescribing drugs, setting broken bones, etc. The soft side is prevention and nutrition, left to "pink collar" professionals like dietitians.

Prevention not "macho" enough

3) ***Minimal money:*** Medical students have to keep their eye on their future, and health insurance companies reimburse very little for nutritional counseling.

How does my doctor decide what to prescribe for me?

Most of the knowledge about the drugs doctors prescribe comes from drug company sales reps, few of whom have any formal training in the subject themselves. So it's like the blind leading the blind. Moreover, drug companies "bribe" doctors with such inducements as frequent flyer miles and "research grants" to use specific drugs.

Proof: As reported in the *Wall Street*

Journal, in 1994 the U.S. Department of Health and Human Services issued a nationwide "Special Fraud Alert" to warn patients of possible illegal marketing tactics by drug companies.

So they prescribe what's lucrative for them rather than what's good for me?

Their hope is that they can do both, but with the rise in "iatrogenic" illness (the creation of new health problems resulting from treatment) that often is not the case. Frankly, it is hard for many doctors to resist the pampering of drug companies, who introduce themselves very early in a doctor's career.

Early bribes: Often, drug companies will provide a medical student's first stethoscope or black bag. During a doctor's low-paying internship and residency, drug companies are known to whisk them off on free vacation weekends in return for attending a seminar on the company's latest drug. And, of course, as the doctor begins to build a practice, the drug companies are right there to provide free business cards, prescription pads and samples.

Drug companies "buy" many doctors during internship

So patients are getting sicker after treatment from their orthodox doctor?

Yes they are. But this is not an indictment of the whole profession. I know many doctors who are dedicated, capable individuals. Still, additional health problems after treatment has become a major problem. In fact, a few startling studies have shown that whenever doctors are NOT on duty, fewer people die.

Death rate drops when docs off duty

Proof: The last time doctors in Los Angeles took to the picket line to protest the high cost of malpractice insurance, the result was an 18% drop in the death rate during this period! In Bogota, Columbia, that same year, striking doctors refused to handle all but emergency cases, and the death rate dropped 35%!!

Reason: Most authorities attribute this phenomenon to the temporary lull in unnecessary surgery and administration of toxic drugs. What makes this situation particularly sad is there is often a highly-effective, natural non-toxic therapy for many such patients. Unfortunately, physicians are either not aware of these alternatives, or chose to ignore them. [I urge you to request my free Special Report, *Naturally Immune for Life* for a directory of safe, non-toxic alternatives to costly Rxs].

How would a physician with an N.D. treat me differently than one with an M.D.?

First, let me explain that a Naturopathic Doctor (N.D.) like myself is clinically trained in the use of natural therapies.

We prefer non-invasive treatments with fewer risks

We don't just treat your symptoms, we try to restore and reinforce your body's natural healing systems with medicines and techniques that are in harmony with natural processes. We much prefer non-invasive treatments that involve fewer risks and side effects.

Do keep in mind: We are not opposed to—and do recommend—the use of surgery or pharmaceuticals for medical problems that our approaches may not be appropriate to treat.

Most important, we consider ourselves teachers as well as physicians. Our aim is to help *you* understand and take more control over factors that effect your health and longevity.

Difference: To many in the M.D. community, you have turned over your power to heal—to them. So in the relatively small amount of time they have to spend with you, even in an initial office visit, all they can do is make a quick diagnosis, write a prescription or recommend a test. Thus, you begin to view yourself as helpless in the face of illness and dependent on them to make you well.

Contrast: A typical first visit to an N.D.

N.D.s take an hour, M.D.s average 7 min. takes an hour—an empowering hour—in which there is a careful assessment of your nutritional balance and consideration of possible lifestyle causes—besides conventional diagnostics. While an M.D. is more likely to emphasize powerful drugs for assaults on disease-causing invaders, an N.D. will likely recommend *drug-sparing* techniques and therapies.

Consider: 85 percent of your illnesses are self-healing and run their natural course. We believe *you,* as an individual, have the power over most of the remaining 15 percent as well, and thus can do more for your good health than any one else.

Ronald Glasser, an *enlightened* M.D. writes, "It is the body that is the hero, not science, not antibiotics . . . not machines or new devices . . . the task of the physician today is what it has always been, to help the body do what it has learned so well to do on its own during its unending struggles for survival—to heal itself."

EASY REMINDERS:

- Medical schools do not train doctors in preventive medicine or nutrition.

- Doctors often count on drug companies for "education."

- Doctors are often bribed to prescribe certain drugs.

- A lot of patients get sick again because of their treatment.

- Naturopathic doctors empower you to heal yourself with nature's own remedies.

CHAPTER 7

Let Me Pause To Tell You the Chilling Story of a Person Very Close to Me.

Ed was his name. *And in April of 1986, he was rushed to the hospital in a small New England community with a heartbeat so irregular—racing and then slowing, racing and then missing a beat—there was a danger it would simply tear itself apart.*

His wife, Marjorie, called me and on the other end of the phone pleaded, "Please help my husband!"

Some of the best cardiologists on the East Coast had put Ed on powerful drugs to control his heart. But the drugs had had the opposite effect. Instead of getting better, Ed was sinking fast.

"He's got a possible liver tumor."

Ed's doctors delivered this chilling prospect to Marjorie, asking her permission to do exploratory surgery or, they said, "Ed may not live another week."

Marjorie was devastated. This was the man she had loved for 40 years of married life. And now her doctors were telling her she was about to lose him. She asked me to come quickly and see what I could do, if anything.

I hopped a red-eye flight that night and arrived at the hospital the next morning. Walking into Ed's room and seeing his condition would have convinced anyone that Ed was very near the end of his life.

He was mentally confused, had double vision and his hands and legs were trembling horribly. There was a terrible bleeding beneath his skin and he was covered with angry bruises.

Ed's body was swollen with fluid.

He had gone almost six weeks without sleep and every part of his bloated body hurt. It was clear to me that Ed was far too sick to go through surgery. Before I left his room, I canceled his surgery, much to the consternation of Ed's doctors. I told them, in no uncertain terms, that I believed Ed was having a life-threatening reaction to the drugs they were giving him.

"You're wrong," sniffed the Cardiologist. "It's not the drug; it's probably the liver tumor and attendant infection."

I told Ed and Marjorie I didn't have all the answers yet, but that I thought I could help Ed get well. This once-robust, now wasted-looking zombie of a man looked at me through glassy eyes. His voice was little more than a hoarse whisper. "I'll do whatever it takes."

I immediately suspended the drug he was taking.

In my professional opinion, there was no earthly reason for Ed to be taking the powerful, potentially-toxic drug the doctors had insisted on. I immediately got him off of it, and started him on several plant-based therapies, plus a change in his nutrition and other naturopathic measures to leech the toxic residue of those drugs out of his system.

And, lo and behold, within a day or two, Ed started taking a turn for the better. Within a week he was thinking more clearly and finally getting some sleep. After two weeks, Ed's bruises had faded and the swelling had gone down. But Ed was still a very sick gentleman. I continued "bathing" his system in a prescribed set of nutrients from nature's pharmacy and he continued to make progress.

One day, his heart suddenly resumed normal functioning.

I was giving Ed a naturopathic manipulation and his heart suddenly returned to its normal sinus rhythm. As soon as that happened, he had more energy than he'd had in years. In fact, he got up and danced a jig on the steps of my clinic!

From then on, Ed got stronger virtually every day. And within a few months, he was a new man. He was smiling again—and so was Marjorie. Her beloved husband's eyes, once faded green-gray, returned to a bright blue. He re-emerged as the vibrant man she knew years ago. We continued to keep his heart rhythm normal using natural therapies, although we knew he would eventually require implantation of a pacemaker to resume an active life. Yet when he finally visited the surgeon who would perform that operation, the doctor couldn't believe his eyes. "Where's the patient?" he asked. "You look too good...in fact you look like a million dollars!" Ed may have been the healthiest patient ever to undergo pacemaker surgery.

A visit to his former doctors

Ed eventually returned to visit the cardiologists who originally treated him. His former doc-

ors were penitent. They agreed their original
reatment had been inappropriate. And although
Ed didn't want to rub it in, he did want to tell the
group they should take a long hard look at their
pill-pushing approach to medicine.

Ed stayed on the natural health lifestyle I'd
given him and kept improving. He led a full,
happy, active life, traveling and visiting friends
all over the country.

Ed's recovery had a very special meaning
for me.

Ed was my dad, Edward Laux—and my best
friend. He passed on not long ago. But for years
after his recovery, Dad encouraged me— urged
me, really—to find a way to reach more than
just the patients I was seeing privately as a
Naturopathic Physician. He said Naturopathy
saved and extended his life, and that he thought I
should share that gift with as many people as are
willing to receive it.

For that reason, I began writing my monthly
Letter, *Naturally Well,* now read by thousands of
people across North America. If you should ever
become a subscriber, you'll appreciate why, on
the back page of the Letter in small print at the
bottom it says, "Dedicated to my dad, Edward
Laux."

CHAPTER 8

The Danger of Antibiotics and What to Take Instead

This is a "wake up call," not meant to *unnecessarily frighten, but to alert you in plenty of time to make some fundamental changes in the way you choose to heal. Antibiotics can be a powerful therapy to many of us, and can continue to be so in times of great need.*

Unfortunately, we are finding that we've relied on that therapy more often than is healthy. And now, instead of healing, instead of boosting our immunity, it's been shown that regular use of antibiotics is more likely to result in our getting sick again, sooner. Indeed, because antibiotics have been prescribed so indiscriminately, they are fast becoming powerless, even dangerous, as the first line of defense against illness.

What is the problem with my using antibiotics?

When you use them to fight a "bug", a small number of the bacteria resist the antibiotic—a natural fact of survival. The trouble is, the resistant bacteria then start to reproduce—at a staggering rate of up to 17 million in 24 hours!

Result: The new bugs are now resistant to the antibiotic you took. So the next time you're ill, you're forced to try a new antibiotic. And that one, too, triggers the growth of resistant bacteria. You get the picture. Before long, when you really need an antibiotic for a life-threatening illness, none may be effective for you.

Fact: In a shocking national survey, seven out of ten people said they occasionally took antibiotics prescribed by their doctor for a cold or flu—illnesses which these drugs have absolutely no effect on.

Are antibiotics only found in drugs I take?

Not by a long shot. The animals we eat are fed some 30 times the total number of antibiotics we take in the U.S. *Thirty times!* These poor cattle, pigs and chickens need

Milk products contain over 80 antibiotics

such heavy dosing because of their nutritionally poor diets and because antibiotics help accelerate the "fattening" process. But in the end, we suffer too. Moreover, processed products from animal sources are just as saturated. Over 80 antibiotics are found in commercial milk, for example. And that's con-

I thought you'd be interested in meeting some of the people who have influenced my life's work, and have benefited from the natural therapies I talk about in this book...

My Family

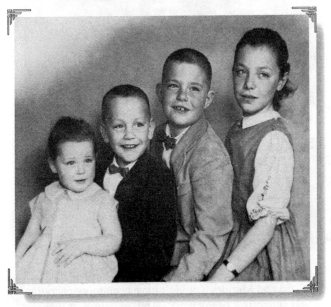

Four Peas in a Pod. All of the Laux kids gravitated into health or environmental fields. (l. to r.) Younger sister Cathy is now an enlightened pharmacist, brother Vern is a naturalist, Me (at age eight), and big sister, Bonnie, is a responsible attorney and environmentalist. We're shown here at home in Wellesley, Massachusetts.

My Parents

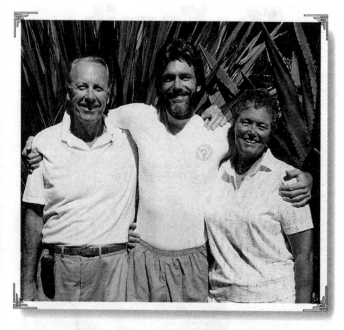

One Proud Son. Everybody should have parents like mine. Ed and Marjorie couldn't have been more encouraging and supportive of my work. And, of course, it may have saved dad's life, as I talk about in this book.

My Dad

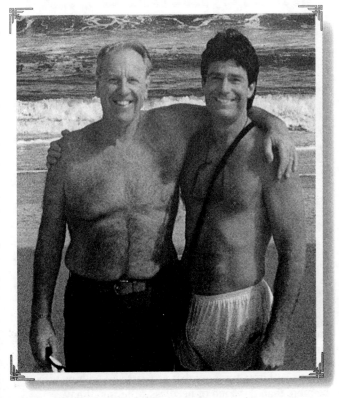

After Dad's Recovery. Here's my dad, Ed, and me back in 1992, several years after his incredible return to good health (see chapter 7). He looks wonderful, doesn't he?

A Day in the Life of a Naturopathic Doctor

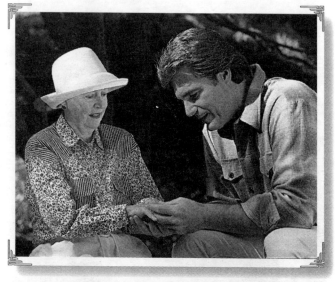

I have ministered to the tender, painful hands and joints of arthritis sufferers for a number of years and nothing affects me more than this kind of needless suffering. I have uncovered a number of very promising natural remedies—one in particular that actually rebuilds cartilage as it reduces swelling—that I discuss in Chapter 10 of this book. I urge you to read it.

TV's Susan Powter invited me on her show to talk about home remedies most of us are not aware of. For example, did you know that one of the great natural remedies for heartburn is eating a banana? It's true. It works as fast as an antacid, but without the risk of getting *rebound* acidity, a recurrence of the problem when the antacid neutralizes too

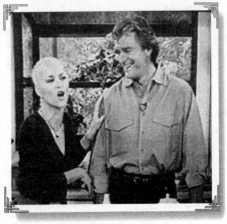

much acid! (Your body then produces more to compensate, so you take more antacid.) You'll find lots of other unexpected—and proven—natural remedies in my monthy Letter, *Naturally Well*.

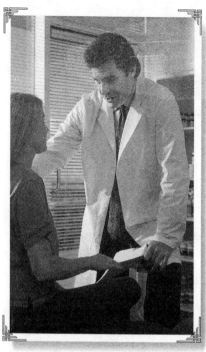

An office visit to a doctor of Natural Medicine is quite a bit different than one to a conventional doctor (see chapter 6). Our evaluation of your health problem and possible solutions are based on many factors, including nutritional, environmental and stress-related considerations and even emotional issues. Chances are, you've never had a conventional doctor evaluate you so thoroughly.

Dr. Laux,

"You have been such a tremendous help to me. So supportive, so generous and so effective. The change in my body's appearance is so exciting. I am stronger in my dance classes than I've been in years. My endurance has increased significantly. My breathing is better and my allergies are under control. My skin is clearer and cleaner. My eyes are bigger and brighter. I am more vital and aware. Any time you need someone to brag about you, I will gladly take the job!"

"The change... is exciting"

Nikki D.

I'm called in to provide consultation on non-drug, non-surgical rehabilitation therapies that speed healing and pain reduction of back problems, migraines, osteoporosis and many other age-related diseases. The point I make to all my patients is that there is so much healing you can do *on your own* without medical intervention.

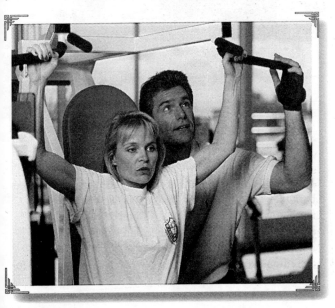

My Expedition to the Amazonian Rainforest

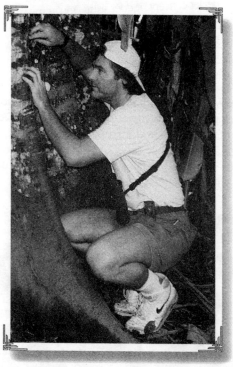

I'm examining one of the many species of medicinal tree bark that, for the Amazonian Indians, is as important as antibiotics are to us. The only difference is that Rainforest "antibiotics" enhance and strengthen your immune system, while excessive use of our synthetic—and often toxic—versions can *compromise* your ability to fight disease (see chapter 8).

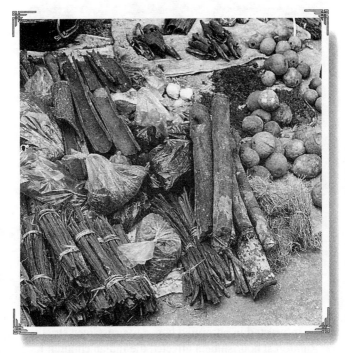

The local Shamans (medicine men) gathered a bounty of natural plants from the Rainforest to show us just a little of the diversity of medicines it yields. There are miracle remedies here that, in just a few short years, will literally shock the world with their incredible healing power.

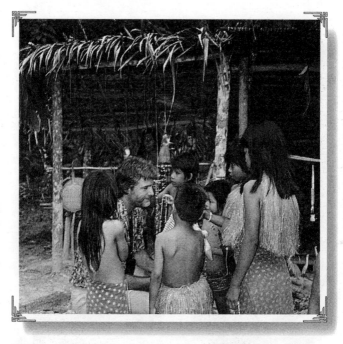

I was interested in observing how a life sustained strictly on Rainforest nourishment affected the Indian children I met. They all exhibited a level of alertness and vitality that—even for healthy children—was remarkable. It's really a lesson for people of any age on the benefits of avoiding our typical high-fat, processes-food lifestyle (see chapter 4).

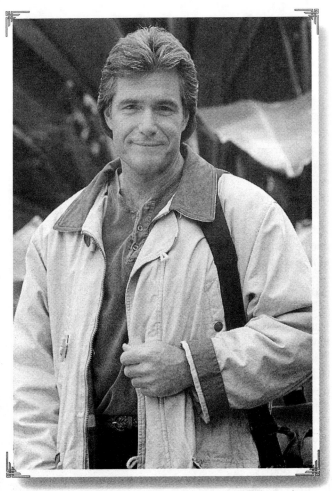

Visiting the "birthplace" of most of the miracle cures the world has known was one of the most rewarding experiences of my life (see chapter 12). And yet would you believe— only 3% of Rainforest species have ever been examined for their medicinal value? I want to help change that.

Inspiring Case Histories

"**I was threatened with cervical cancer at age 31**", confides Amy Tomer. "I had one operation to remove pre-cancerous cells and later my gynecologist wanted me to have another. With the help of Dr. Laux, I discovered that some of the foods I was eating were actually blocking my body's 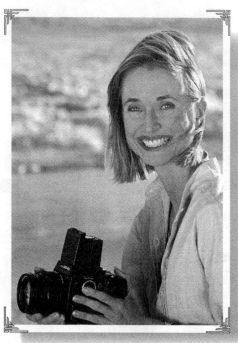 natural healing processes (see chapters 4 & 5). I changed my diet and started taking immune-enhancing nutrients and then opted for the second surgery. Not long after, I had a pap smear and it was completely normal! I'm living proof that Dr. Laux's approach works."

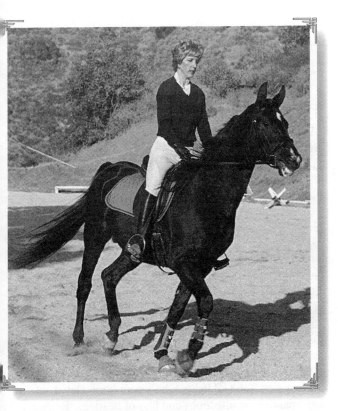

"I was so sick of being sick" says bookkeeper, Debbie Mickelson. "After my seventh surgery in 24 years, somebody told me about Dr. Laux. I followed his program of nutrition to pump up my immune system and followed his advice on how to handle stress (see chapter 11). It worked! At 44, people tell me I look ten years younger!"

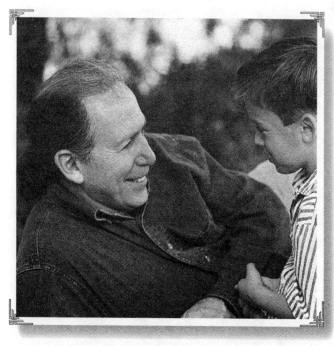

"We were told surgery was our son's only hope," recalls store owner, Bob Goldberg, who's young son David suffered painful ear infections and loss of hearing. "But we decided to get a second opinion—from Dr. Laux. We learned that chronic ear infections are often brought on by food allergies. After testing, it turned out he was right. It was like a miracle! Within a month, David's ears cleared!"

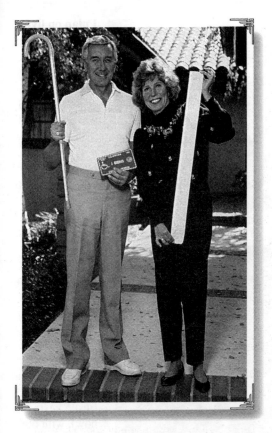

"My arthritis was so bad, I couldn't even shake hands", remembers Bob Kazmirski, a retired insurance executive. "My doctor prescribed a *chemotherapy* drug with a three foot long list of side effects (my wife is holding). Plus, I had to endure painful cortisone shots. All that, and the arthritis kept getting worse. That's when I decided to give Dr. Laux's approach a try (see chapter 10). His program changed my life! In three weeks the pain was completely gone. I no longer need my cane or disabled license plate. My only regret is that I waited so long to try the Laux approach."

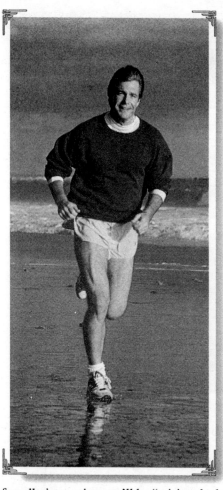

I plan on living to be 120 along with you. Here's why: At the beginning of the century, age 60 was considered "old age"—now it's considered merely the youth of old age. In the 1950's, you were old at age 75— yet now, 75-year old adults lead extremely active, robust lives. But between 1960 and 1990, people leading vigorous lives beyond age 85 became com- mon-place. And by the year 2000 (just 5 years from now), with our knowledge of the biological and nutritional secrets of longevity pro- foundly increasing, we'll be "raising the bar" again, to more than 100 year old. So it's very easy to project that in the years ahead, living to be a healthy 110-120 years will become almost routine. The best part is—it doesn't take a lot of sacrifice to aim for it. I'll help you stay on that road every month in *Naturally Well*.

sidered an officially "safe" level. Yet such levels have accelerated the emergence of resistant bacteria by nearly 3000%!

Result: You could be consuming milk, cheese, yogurt and butter tainted with antibiotics and drug-resistant bugs. A good reason to buy organically-produced milk at your local health food store.

So what can I do to protect myself when I must take antibiotics for illness?

At the very least, re-inoculate yourself with life-supporting bacteria by using a supplement that contains friendly bacteria like acidophilus. Use as directed during your antibiotic prescription, and for three weeks thereafter. I use a product called Inner Ecology from Prevail. It's available at most health food stores.

How can I stay healthy without taking drugs or antibiotics?

Begin taking nature's own antibiotics—herbs. They "pump up" your immune system as nothing else can, enabling your body to take on all enemies, foreign and domestic. If your immune system is strong, it can easily repel most bugs, viruses and other invaders to keep you in robust good health and promote longevity. When your underlying immune response is not operating properly, even antibiotics are useless.

How do specific herbs work to charge up my immune system?

Herbs have been consumed as potent health-giving plants for thousands of years. And they've been extremely effective. In fact, a number of today's prescription drugs as well as over-the-counter remedies are based on herbal and plant medicine.

Examples: Digitalis, the heart drug is taken from the foxglove plant...aspirin comes from the bark of the white willow tree...Penicillin comes from a mold first used by ancient Egyptians 4,000 years ago...Ben-Gay and Vicks Vaporub use herbal ingredients.

Difference: Many pharmaceuticals taken from natural medicine only use a "blueprint" of the original active ingredient, which is then turned into a synthetic and patented. It contains none of the natural buffers inherent in the original plant, which is one reason why there can be so many dangerous drug side effects.

Drugs get their "blueprint" from herbs

What are some of the most beneficial herbs I can use right now?

I'd start off with these three just to show you the remarkable ability of herbs to enhance your immune mechanisms:

1. *Echinacea,* from the purple coneflower, was used by the American Indian as a blood purifier and snake bite remedy. (Those are Echinacea flowers I'm pictured with on the cover.) This herb has now shown to significantly enhance your immune system's efforts in neutralizing viruses, destroying bacteria and rushing white blood cells to an infection site.

2. *Goldenseal* is an herb native to eastern North America that is very effective against "staph" infections* and "strep" and salmonella bacteria. It also increases the blood supply to your spleen, an integral part of your immune system. (Goldenseal and Echinacea are also sold in a combination form that gives you double the healing clout.)

3. *Licorice Root* has been used in both western and eastern cultures for several thousand years. It has potent anti-viral effects and it is very effective for treating respiratory tract infections like bronchitis and pneumonia. It is also a great cold medication if used three

times a day in capsule form.

[NOTE: There are so many medicinal herbs to choose from that I have included a special directory of many effective ones in *Naturally Immune for Life*. See the back of this book for ordering information]

EASY REMINDERS:

- Regular use of antibiotics is likely to make you sick again sooner.

- They are prescribed indiscriminately by doctors unaware of effective natural cures.

- You are also getting regularly dosed with antibiotics through the meat that you eat.

- Start using nature's own antibiotics—herbs.

- Echinacea, Goldenseal and Licorice Root are good herbs to start with.

---

*I always delight in observing someone discover the healing power of herbs for the first time, and that happened during the writing of this book. My editor, Jerry Fisher, complained of a nagging scalp infection he'd been fighting for many months without success. (Unfortunately, he was trying to beat it with antibiotics prescribed by his doctor and it was having little effect.) I suggested he try Goldenseal for a few weeks and see what happened. He took the advice and, sure enough, his first experience in taking one of nature's antibiotics resulted in the complete disappearance of his problem.

CHAPTER 9

If Alternative Treatments Work Why Don't You Hear More About Them?

Behind closed doors, the medical establishment has put extreme pressure on alternative therapies and the professionals who practice them. "Sadly my profession is guilty of a bad attitude and even worse behavior toward colleagues who adopt drug-sparing therapies," laments James Carter M.D., author of Racketeering in Medicine, The Suppression of Alternatives, "Natural techniques have helped heal chronic illness throughout the 19th and 20th Centuries with a degree of success about which sometimes the finest of medical specialists can only dream."

Why does the Medical Establishment want to suppress alternative treatments?

In a nutshell, to force conformity in medicine and protect themselves from the competition of doctors using less costly alternatives... alternatives that often cancel the need for surgery and drugs.

How do I know if my doctor is involved?

Actually, few doctors in practice are even aware of these behind-the-scenes maneuvers. And it must be told that there are a few who secretly recommend alternative treatments, but warn their patients never to breath a word of it for fear of getting in trouble.

Are there any valuable treatments, beside medications, I might be deprived of because of this?

Chelation therapy is a major one I've talked about in my monthly Letter. It's a simpler, safer way of unclogging your arteries and veins of dead-

How to gain "younger" arteries without surgery

ly plaque—thus avoiding costly (and sometimes dangerous) bypass surgery or angioplasty. Instead, you achieve arterial clearing through an IV injection of a very safe amino acid, EDTA. This treatment also removes calcium build-up that results from the aging process. So you end up with "younger" arteries in several ways.

What has been the success rate of this therapy?

It's estimated that some 80% of patients submitting to chelation therapy are significantly helped. And a great many have avoided expensive bypass and angioplasty surgery in the process. There are numerous cases on record in which severely impaired patients are now leading normal, robust lives thanks to chelation.

If it's that successful, why doesn't Big Medicine simply adopt it for its own?

In a word, profit. Chelation costs about $3,000 to perform compared to $30,000-50,000 for a bypass procedure. Chelation is performed humbly in a doctor's office without the need for a hospital, a surgeon, a cardiologist, an anesthesiologist or the rest of the army of professionals that pocket the health-care billions bankrupting this country. There is hope, however, because the FDA has just recently approved Chelation for testing.

Yes, but might I still need and benefit from bypass and angioplasty?

It's possible, but even the American Medical Association admitted that nearly 50% of all bypass surgery is performed for the wrong rea-

son. I've seen estimates as high as 85% of
bypass patients who don't meet the criteria for
benefit.

Result: Bypass surgery—a $10 million-a-day
industry—manages to reduce
Make out your the population by some
will before you 28,000 patients annually.
try it Angioplasty is a $4 billion
business and sends nearly
9,000 patients a year to an early grave.

Is the on-going attack on supplements part of the same harassment?

You bet it is. The medical establishment has
spent the last 50 years trying to suppress vitamins, minerals and herbs in order to convince
the public that expensive, toxic drugs and dangerous surgery are the only possible remedies.

Reason: Since natural medicines from plant
sources cannot be patented, drug companies—
who can mark up their patented pills up to
3000%—are not interested. And they obviously
don't want you to be interested in them either.
That's why they continue to discredit them in
any way, even if it means spreading misinforma-
tion.

[NOTE: Despite the harassment, people need
to know about these alternatives. That's why I

write my monthly Letter
Naturally Well. If you
wish, you can request a
subscription at the end
of this book.]

**Drug companies
only sanction cures
they can patent**

EASY REMINDERS:

- The medical establishment protects its profits
  by denouncing practitioners offering less
  expensive, non-invasive procedures.

- Chelation has proven its ability to unclog
  arteries, yet is denounced by conventional
  medicine.

- Traditional bypass costs 10 times more than
  chelation—at 100 times the risk.

- Bypass is a $10 million A DAY industry.

- Supplements are discredited because drug
  companies can't patent them.

CHAPTER 10

Pain Relief That's NOT What Your Doctor Orders

Never take aspirin for arthritis or any nonsteroid anti-inflammatory drug (NSAIDs)— like Motrin, Advil or Nuprin—that a conventional doctor might recommend. They may decrease your pain in the short run, but worsen your condition in the long run by stopping new cartilage formation and increasing cartilage destruction.

Worst of all, the dosage required to suppress your symptoms can cause life-threatening peptic ulcers (as evidenced by the hospitalization in Canada of Secretary of State, Warren Christopher, who was taking NSAIDS for arthritis). According to Michael Murray, author of the acclaimed book, Natural Alternatives to Over-The-Counter and Prescription Drugs *"more people die each year as a result of peptic ulcers caused by NSAIDs than from cocaine abuse." And it almost goes without saying that high-potency prescription drugs can have even greater side-effect consequences.*

Is there any good news for arthritis pain sufferers?

Yes, and the good news is twofold. First, you should know that arthritis can actually disappear on its own, without any treatment. That can be

_____

Hip pain can greatly improve without treatment

_____

bittersweet news if you've been enduring arthritis pain for some time. But one long-term study of patients with advanced osteoarthritis showed that after 10 years of no treatment, about 50% of affected hip joints improved dramatically. So, never underestimate your power to self heal.

The second bit of news is (and by this point in the book, you may already suspect) that arthritis can be positively affected by lifestyle, diet, supplements and other natural health care practices.

Proof: In a research study involving 250,000 arthritis patients conducted by Robert Bingham M.D., some 85% reported substantial relief through the use of nutritional supplements.

What medicine should I take beyond what my doctor says?

Nature's best remedy: Today there's a remarkable (and SAFE) all-natural supplement called Glucosamine Sulfate that actually reverses arthritis, helping your body rebuild cartilage and reduce joint tenderness and swelling. So where NSAIDs only offer relief from symptoms and may actually encourage the disease process, Glucosamine Sulfate supplements address the cause of the disease. Take one capsule three times a day with meals. Available from Enzymatic Therapy (800) 783-2286, among other makers.

I could fill a book on all the arthritis relievers recommended to me. Is there something utterly simple I can take?

You mean you haven't heard about crocodile droppings, frog sperm and earthworm oil? (Those were actual recommendations years ago.) Stop by the drug store and pick up some ordinary cod liver oil. Research has shown that taking fish oil capsules (containing omega-3 fatty acids) results in much less joint pain and

Natural no-side-effect relief exists

fatigue. But instead of paying a premium for fancy fish oil capsules, just buy that old standby derived from the friendly cod. (Vegetarian alternative: Flaxseed oil.)

Extra benefit: Cod liver oil is also rich in bone-building vitamin D and inflammation-fighting vitamin A.

What foods should I avoid?

Since arthritis is not nearly as common in societies that stress a diet of natural whole foods, and that de-emphasize sugar and saturated fat, it suggests that this should be your healing meal plan.

Aggravators: I recommend you also stay clear of nuts and nut products like peanut butter. Also avoid refined sugars, fried foods, alcohol, tobacco, coffee and drugs. The same goes for margarine, shortening and refined or hydrogenated cooking or salad oils. Yes, it's a stringent list—but you'll be ridding yourself of some of the worst aggravators of arthritis.

Some say stay away from the "nightshade" family of foods. Why?

It does sound a little contradictory, I know, since nightshade foods include normally health-ful veggies like tomatoes, potatoes, eggplant and red peppers. But some years back, a researcher named Norman Childers announced a nightshade-free diet that cured his osteoarthritis and it's been given credence ever since.

Not all veggies are kind to your joints

Reason: If you're genetically-prone to arthritis, you might bring on its onset through long-term, low-level consumption of alkaloids found in those vegetables. Alkaloids may inhibit normal collagen repair in joints or cause inflammation.

Proof: Dr. Childers conducted a study of some 5,000 arthritis patients who agreed to avoid nightshade variety vegetables for a prescribed period of time. More than 70% reported relief from aches and pains. Pretty convincing proof.

Are there supplements that help the healing?

Yes. In fact, antioxidant supplements are vitally important to your battle against arthritis because they bombard the free-radical invaders that are the direct cause of arthritis.

So "up" your intake of vitamin E to 800 i.u. a day, vitamin C to 3 to 5 grams a day and also vitamin B6 to 50 mg—all have been found to help reduce inflammation and, ultimately, pain.

Earlier in this book I also introduced you to green superfoods as a smart supplement for treating arthritis.

Here's why: Green superfoods (such as spirulina, Chlorella, wheat grass, barley grass or alfalfa) detoxify and bring about a level of "inner ecology" in your body. It is in this environment that your immune system can be the most productive in repairing joint damage.

What about chronic back pain—do I just have to "live with it"?

No—and I'm a good example of how to overcome it. Years ago I broke my back playing football. After that, I had low back and disc problems and everything from mild discomfort to intense, sharp burning pain. Sound familiar?

I've had severe sciatica in both legs down to my heels. I couldn't stand up straight for weeks at a time, and I had to support myself on whatever was around me wherever I moved. Just getting out of bed was a monumental achievement. And sitting for a period of time or driving a car was, at times, unbearable. So I know your pain. I know your limitations. But, my back problems are ancient history thanks to some special measures I took.

My severe back pain is now ancient history

What kinds of actions did you take that I can adapt for myself?

The first is to make yourself aware that you don't have a "bad back." To buy into that notion gives your back power over you instead of the other way around. You have a back that is sending you signals of a kind of distress that you can do something about.

Chiropractic and acupuncture are the best outside remedies for overcoming back pain (see chapter 13 for the benefits of each). But one self-administered relief technique that I found very beneficial involves laying on a device called a MA-Roller, which is a piece of wood lathed like a chair leg so that the wide areas can go on either side of your spine. (It's available in health food stores.) Lay on the floor and place it under your lower back—or wherever you have a problem. Rest and relax on it.

Result: It provides strong trigger point stimulus and muscle relaxation.

The Ball Method: If you can't find a MA-Roller, buy and use an ordinary tennis ball for lower back or hip pain. Lying on the floor, place the ball directly under— or as near as can be endured to—the area of pain. In a matter of a few minutes, you'll likely feel

Self-administered pinpoint pressure does the job

less pain in the areas receiving the pressure. Treatment to any given area shouldn't last more than fifteen minutes.

Are there any headache remedies that don't require me to pop a pill?

Yes—some effective ones. But let me say first how right you are to look beyond the medicine cabinet. As I write this book, research has only recently been released that claims taking more than one tablet each day of today's most popular headache reliever—Acetaminophen, largely sold as Tylenol—doubles your risk of kidney failure. In another study released at the same time, Tylenol was also shown as a threat to cause serious liver damage if consumed in quantity on an empty stomach.

No warning: Many people have been taking Acetaminophen regularly on the assumption that, if there was a problem, they would have been warned by the medical establishment. Not a good assumption. And because many were switched to Acetaminophen from an equally-risky painkiller, aspirin, the question is: What and who can you trust to relieve severe pain without potentially lethal consequences?

What CAN you trust?

Medicinal herbs, such as willow bark, scullcap, feverfew, Jamaican dogwood, rosemary or valerian (available at your local health food store) are quite effective for occasional headaches.

Without swallowing anything: Here are a few measures that can offer fast headache relief:

Thumbs up: Press your thumb against the roof of your mouth firmly for about five minutes. Try to center it under the location of the headache. It can give you relief.

Acupressure: Hold your thumb and forefinger firmly together and then with your other thumb press firmly on the mound that forms between them on the back of your hand. This action can provide pain relief. You can also get relief by pressing directly above the inner corner of the eye or against the bone that forms the top of the eye socket.

Touch relief: Lie down, close your eyes, and have someone lightly touch parts of your body, moving from the shoulders down to the toes. Acknowledge each touch with a simple "okay."

You CAN take control of headache pain

The purpose is to move you away from concentrating on the pain in your head and get you back in touch with the rest of your body. This technique is also very effective for a head cold.

EASY REMINDERS:

- Don't take aspirin or any NSAID for arthritis pain. It can cause long-term joint damage.

- Arthritis can actually disappear on its own, or improve dramatically without treatment.

- Nature's best remedy is Glucosamine Sulfate, which actually reverses arthritis, helping to rebuild cartilage.

- Stay clear of saturated fats (meat and dairy), refined sugars, fried foods, alcohol, tobacco, coffee and drugs.

- Experiment with avoidance of "nightshade" foods.

- Take Green Superfoods to enhance the healing environment for arthritis.

- Use the roller or ball method of relieving back pain.

- Don't take Tylenol regularly for headache pain—it may cause kidney and liver damage, among other problems.

- Use herbs and/or body work to make the pain go away.

CHAPTER 11

Your Secret Weapon Against Aging: Your Mind.

Listen to Franz Alexander M.D.: "The fact that the mind rules the body is, in spite of its neglect by biology and medicine, the most fundamental fact we know about the process of life." (Yet another conventional doctor who's seen the light.) In truth, there is an intimate two-way communication system between your mind and your body's immune system. It's a pipeline through which your emotions can affect your body's ability to heal itself, defend itself and preserve itself.

Is there actual proof that what I'm thinking or feeling is affecting my immune system?

I know of a fascinating little experiment that proved it in the simplest way: Volunteers were injected with a small dose of adrenaline—just enough to produce the same reaction in you as if someone jumped out of the shadows and yelled "boo."

Result: Immediate blood tests showed an

instant decline in protective white blood cells, revealing the effect that the feeling of fear had on the immune system.

Does this show I can strengthen or weaken my immunities with certain emotions?

You bet. Your thoughts and emotions stimulate or depress your immune system, which has a direct effect on how resistant you are to the bacteria, viruses and microbes in your life. So even though you're not consciously aware of it or in conscious control, your mind can make you sick tomorrow and it can also keep you well until age 120.

Could I eat right and exercise regularly and still "kick the bucket" prematurely?

It happens. Let anger, frustration, fear or other negative emotions dominate your mind, and it will depress your immune system, making you more susceptible to sickness.

Even marathon runners have died prematurely

Example: The lack of human companionship through death or divorce can produce feelings of loneliness and isolation that are one of the leading causes of premature death.

Can I protect myself from specific diseases by addressing specific emotions?

Yes. It's been proven, for example, that prolonged hostility causes excessive secretion of norepinephrine—a stress hormone—which contributes to your risk of high blood pressure, arteriosclerosis or a heart attack. If you can avoid such stresses, you can sustain strong immunities against many killer diseases.

[NOTE: I reveal other connections between specific emotions you feel and the illness they cause, plus how to overcome them, in my complimentary Special Report *Naturally Immune for Life*. See the end of this book for ordering information.]

Are there any natural "magic bullets" for stress?

Actually, there is a class of stress-reducing herbs that I feel approach "magic bullet" status. They're called adaptogenic herbs and they can have a dramatic effect on normalizing, even optimizing, your ability to handle mental and physical stress. Not only that, they are freely available, over-the-counter non-drug wonders!

The #1 Adaptogen: Siberian Ginseng is the anti-fatigue, anti-stress herb *par excellence*. It can also improve your overall health and vitality, increase your longevity and sharpen your memory to boot! (NOTE: Siberian Ginseng is best used in a 60-day regimen. After that, give it a rest until you again feel the need for help during a particularly stressful period.)

Sample its effectiveness free of charge

Best of all: If you'd like to sample the effectiveness of Siberian Ginseng free of charge, just to see what a positive effect it can have, see the back of this book for special details.

How do I deal with the causes of stress, to keep them from ultimately affecting my health?

You might start with a simple three-minute Stress Test I've developed that could keep this silent assassin from being a threat to your health. [It's part of the Special Report mentioned earlier] Here's why:

Stress breaks down your body and ages you like few other influences. If you can neutralize some of the causes by confronting them in ways I suggest, you've taken a giant step toward stress reduction—and healthful longevity.

Breaking point: The body can usually handle a single large stressful event, just as a piece of metal can withstand a strong force and not break. But chronic stress, equivalent to bending that piece of metal back and forth, over and over, IS going to "break" your health. That

Stress reduction leads to a longer life

continuous strain and tension is obviously what you want—and need—to avoid.

What's the real skinny on laughter, and how it can effect my health?

For at least a generation, the Reader's Digest has published a regular feature called "Laughter is the Best Medicine." You've probably chuckled at it yourself. But I doubt the editors had the scientific back-up for that title when the feature first appeared. They do today.

Reason: Research has shown that laughter and other positive emotions rally the body's natural defenses against stress, pain and disease. In fact, the study of humor and its effects on the body even has a name. It's called Gelotology. A Stanford University professor and well-known Gelotologist has written that, besides increasing heart rate and hormone production, laughter moves extra nutrients and oxygen into your body's tissues. This combination, in effect, bathes tensed, stressed or troubled areas of the body in a healing balm.

What about meditation as a stress eraser—it gets poo-poo'd as something only Zen monks do?

Meditation is misunderstood by a great many people. It is an utterly simple exercise of the mind that can have rather powerful results. And it is practiced by people in all walks of life, from the butcher to the baker to, yes, the Zen monk. Moreover, it may well be the ultimate stress eraser, because it produces a psychological state of deep relaxation much different and more satisfying than that achieved from just sleep or rest.

Biological reaction: Independent research studies have shown that when you meditate, the lactate concentration in

Tension drops 4 times faster than thru resting

your blood (related to anxiety and tension) decreases sharply, nearly four times as fast as when you are simply resting quietly. Proof of a uniquely-relaxed state.

Skin Test: In a landmark study to determine the actual level (or deepness) of relaxation achieved through meditation, researchers did something interesting. They applied a micro-electric current to the skin of meditators, a practice well known for indicating the amount of tension and anxiety present. The more tension, the ower the resistance to the current. The less tension, the higher the resistance.

Results: The study showed that during meditation, skin resistance increased as much as 400%!

Why would my body respond this way?

Meditation is a practice in which your mind is focused on doing just one thing—and that's simply the act of meditating. Since your mind is accustomed to being extremely busy with thoughts and feelings—

> **Deep relaxation comes by doing just one thing**

even while you're sleeping or resting—doing just one thing is a comparatively relaxed mode.

Lawrence LeShan in *How to Meditate* describes it as follows:

> *"If you think about the signals we are sending to ourselves at most times in our daily life, we see that they are (many). If I am talking to someone, I am usually not only talking. I am also thinking about where the conversation is going, what has already been said, how I feel about the person I am communicating with and what the time is. In addition I am conscious of my posture, the feelings of my body, my fatigue level*

*and the people who may be moving
around near me. By contrast, in meditation, we are sending only one set of signals."*

Would you like a simple way to try out meditation for yourself? I offer you an easy method
for getting started in my Special Report,
Naturally Immune for Life.

EASY REMINDERS:

- Your mind can heal you, keep you healthy and
  help you live longer.

- Your mind can also affect you negatively,
  depressing your immune system and making
  you more susceptible to illness.

- A special 3-minute self test helps you start on
  the road to freedom from stress.

- Laughter is among the best medicines for
  stress.

- Meditation is misunderstood by a lot of people
  and offers uniquely-beneficial relaxation.

CHAPTER 12

What I Discovered in the Amazonian Rainforest, Nature's Richest "Pharmacy."

I saw butterflies bigger than our birds in this beautiful, incredibly complex repository of the world's most powerful natural curatives. The Rainforest is a naturopath's paradise...a botanical treasure of medicinal promise and potential, growing in soil uncorrupted by pesticides and pollution. And it covers more than a billion acres stretching across areas of Brazil, Venezuela, Columbia and parts of Ecuador and Peru. I went as part of an expedition co-sponsored by the American Botanical Counsel and appropriately called, "Pharmacy From the Rain Forest". The purpose was to reconnect with the origins of many of the healing substances that come from Mother Earth. And what I discovered will be very valuable for you to know.

Why is medicine from Rainforest plants so important to me?

Because these plants contain phytochemical defenses more highly evolved than perhaps anywhere else on earth.

Result: The struggle of so many species to survive and even thrive in such a competitive environment has resulted in deeply developed, highly sophisticated armament against attackers of every kind. Research has shown that these extremely potent defenses are also medicinally valuable to human beings for the same preventive reasons. But then, the shamans (medicine men) like those I met in Peru have known this for thousands of years.

What did you learn from the shamans (medicine men) of the Rainforest?

A lot. They reinforced my belief that the best doctor is merely a channel and a guide to the healing power of nature. That is the function they see themselves providing.

I also found them to be a very sharing, very humble fraternity, and yet as wise and learned in their field as any healing professional in our culture. They know the power of these species well, especially how they need to be used to maximize their potency and power. It is said that each time a medicine man from the Rainforest dies, it is as if a library of natural sciences has burned to the ground.

What's an example of a Rainforest species that has become "medicinally valuable" to me?

There are many, but a major one that comes to mind is the Rosy Periwinkle. Some time ago, scientists found that this delicate flower con-

A powerful cure for Hodgkin's disease

tains two powerful alkaloids which have proven to be the most effective cures we know for two particularly deadly cancers, Hodgkin's disease and acute lymphocytic leukemia.

Result: Thanks to derivatives of the Rosy Periwinkle, survival rates for these two killers have gone from 2% to 58% and from 20% to 80% respectively.

Has this encouraged a lot of new research in the Rainforest?

Less than you would imagine. Of more than 250,000 known species in the Rainforest, less than 3% have been tested for their medicinal applications. *And yet out of that 3% has come more than 25% of all the medicines we take!* So

_____

**Bulldozers are
leveling this
delicate ecosystem**

_____

we'd better pick up the pace, because as most people know, the destruction of these delicate ecosystems is well underway. Chainsaws and bulldozers are slowly but surely clearing the way for "civilization".

Are there powerful cures not widely known outside the Rainforest?

Yes, a number of them. But one that may deserve special mention is an herb called Uña de Gato (Cat's Claw). To my mind, the many healing properties of this plant make it destined for identification as a miracle herb in years ahead. The famed Rainforest researcher, Nicole Maxwell, referred to it as "perhaps the most important plant in the Rainforest." And just last year, an unprecedented 2-day National Congress on Uña de Gato was called by the government of Peru to address issues concerning the harvesting of this treasure.

Its origin: Uña de Gato grows as a woody vine in the highlands of the Peruvian Amazon. It has been used for hundreds, perhaps thousands, of years by the native Ashanica Indians who have little access to modern health care.

Uña de Gato is regarded as a powerful and versatile infection fighter and immunity booster. It is used routinely to treat ulcers, gastric disorders, Crohn's disease, genital

Most important plant in the Rainforest

herpes, acne, colitis, hemorrhoids—all, of course, with zero side effects.

Plaque inhibitor: Research on Uña de Gato has also isolated an alkaloid considered likely to reduce the risk of strokes and heart attacks. It has been shown to inhibit the formation of plaque in the arteries and blood clots in the vessels of your brain and heart.

Cancer treatment: Beyond the herb's "routine" powers, Nicole Maxwell reports interviewing cancer patients whose use of Uña de Gato resulted in documented remission of the disease and relief from the side effects of chemotherapy.

Future cure for arthritis, diabetes?
Maxwell further reports: "I learned that a man whose lung cancer was cured by Uña de Gato had, after continued dosage, found that he could walk normally and even climb stairs, although for years he had been badly crippled by arthritis. (I also) got good evidence of it having worked wonders for diabetes."

One "disadvantage": Although Maxwell

used Uña de Gato herself to get rid of a stubborn
infection contracted in the wild, she noted the
following 'side-effect': "After the infection was
beaten, I kept taking Uña de Gato because there
was a lot of flu going around. I didn't get the flu

**Side benefit: It May
return gray hair to
natural color**

but I began to notice an
occasional dark hair (of
her original hair color)
showing up among my
snowy white ones that

I'd been so vain about. And a few more every
week or so. That was disturbing... even though
some might consider it a boon."

**I've always heard of aphrodisiacs in the wild.
Do they really exist—and how credible are
they?**

It's a good question because most of us hear
all the claims about supposed aphrodisiacs—
from bear gallbladders to the scent of cinnamon
buns. The only proven aphrodisiac that herbally-
aware people are conscious of is derived from
the bark of an African tree (Yohimbe). But
Yohimbe, while effective for some men, has a
spotty record of success. Plus, the side effects—
anxiety, panic attacks, dizziness and
headaches—can be, to say the least, a major dis-
traction.

Rainforest alternative: Research that I've

seen, as well as individuals I spoke with on my trip, indicate that an herb called Marapauma (derived from a shrub native to Brazil) may provide better results than Yohimbe but without any side effects.

Proof: In a study by French researcher, Dr. Jacque Waynberg, a renowned authority on sexual dysfunction, 262 patients expressing a lack of sexual desire or "erection failures" were given a daily dose of 1 to 1.5 grams of

At least one in every two men gets results

Marapauma. Within two weeks, 62% of those claiming a loss of libido said that treatment definitely had a positive effect. 52% of those with erection problems also felt that Marapauma had helped them.

Are there other unique Rainforest herbs I should know about?

There are a whole range of plant-based remedies from this region that effectively treat everything from headache to high blood pressure to gout to insomnia—naturally and non-toxically. As a result, there have been a number of volumes written on Rainforest medicines. But for those who would prefer to read more of a concise digest of the most proven and effective of these herbs, I have only recently produced another Special Report, *Cures From The Rainforest Pharmacy* now being made available from my publisher free to subscribers of my Letter, *Naturally Well.*

   Bonus: Through special arrangement with a U.S. importer of Rainforest herbs, new subscribers to my Letter may also immediately receive free samples of both Uña de Gato and Marapauma. It's an unique opportunity to experience these miracle substances for yourself without cost. See the back of this book or the enclosed order form for further details.

EASY REMINDERS:

- Plant-based medicine from the Rainforest contain perhaps the most powerful disease-fighting phytochemicals on earth.

- The Rosy Periwinkle contains alkaloids that are now effectively used for treatment of two deadly cancers.

- Uña de Gato (Cat's Claw) may be the most important herb in the Rainforest; a powerful infection fighter and immunity booster.

- Marapauma is a bona fide aphrodisiac without side effects.

- Other Rainforest herbs treat headache, high blood pressure, etc.

CHAPTER 13

Potent Natural Remedies You Should Know More About

You NEED to know about Naturopathic alternatives...no matter how you decide to address a health issue in your life. Even if you ultimately choose a more conventional approach to prevention or treatment, you MUST be aware of the natural, non-toxic, alternative before making a final decision. That's why I created my monthly Letter, Naturally Well. To give you a balanced perspective for some of the most important decisions in your life.

All the topics you've read about so far in this little book are among the subjects I regularly update in Naturally Well, plus all the following...

✔ *The Weight Loss Breakthrough You've Been Waiting For:* The term "breakthrough" is often used indiscriminately, but it is entirely justified when applied to a safe, non-toxic, non-addictive derivative of an Asian fruit, Garcinia cambogia. The orange-sized fruit has traditionally been used for, among other things, a spice in curries. But Brandeis University researchers discovered that an extract of Garcina, hydroxycitric acid (HCA), can be a godsend to the overweight individual.

3 powerful benefits:

1) Its unique chemistry effectively reduces your appetite, and thus your food intake

2) It actually stems fat production from the foods you do eat

3) While it's doing all that, it also increases your energy level.

The optimal dose of hydroxycitric acid has yet to be determined, but a good starting point is one to two gram doses an hour before meals. Also *there is no weight rebound effect if you stop taking it!* There is much more exciting information yet to come out on HCA and I will update you in *Naturally Well* as these final pieces of this exciting solution are in place.

Curry spice may be a weight loss miracle

[Meanwhile, if you'd like to experience the marvelous benefits of HCA with a free sample, see the back of this book for details.]

✔ How To Make Depression Go Away, Naturally

Are you sometimes tempted to take one of those mood-altering drugs to artificially raise your spirits? Wait. Researchers are leaning more and more toward the theory that feelings of depression can quite often have a nutritional cause. Think about it: if your mind can affect your body, your body may also affect your mind. Certain nutrient deficiencies can be causing or contributing to your depression.

Examples: 1) Many cases of depression have been greatly improved—or even cured—when the person's folic acid levels were normalized. (Folic Acid deficiency is the most common nutritional deficiency in the world.) *2)* A Vitamin B-6 deficiency can

Your depression may be nutrition-related

bring about a depressed state because it reduces the level of serotonin—a mood elevator—in your brain. These are just two of many possible nutritional causes for depression I now touch on regularly in *Naturally Well.*

Possible breakthrough: The closest thing to a natural wonder drug—no side effects, no toxicity—for depression may be a substance called tyrosine. In an initial pilot study, subjects reported a 60%-70% improvement in mood, a rate comparable to most major antidepressants. I promise to keep you posted on further important refinements in this very promising therapy.

✔ "Fix" Your Bad Back by Passing Gas.

No joke. However, the gas I'm referring to is that which is released from your joint fluid during a painless chiropractic manipulation. Chiropractic treatment, the preference of millions of people each year for non-toxic, non-surgical pain relief, involves thrusting maneuvers in which a joint is stretched to just beyond its normal range of movement, producing a painless click or crack as the joint gases are released.

Experience a wave of relaxation

Results: What typically follows is a wave of relief and relaxation.

Improvement from this therapy can range from gradual to oftentimes dramatic so natural functioning is restored. It is based on the concept that realignment of your spine sends a healing directive (via your nervous system) to the trouble spot. I regularly introduce you to specific chiropractic solutions to your health needs in *Naturally Well*.

✔ How To Get Sustained Pain Relief From Regular "Needling"

I'm speaking, of course, about acupuncture, the once scoffed at, now widely-embraced form of healing that originated in the Orient thousands of years ago. Acupuncture involves the usually painless insertion of very fine needles (designed to push your skin fibers apart rather than cut)

Healing energy is sent to the area of pain

along energy channels in your body—called meridians. According to the Chinese, this process re-balances the "chi" or life force in your body, which, when thrown out of balance, can cause illness and disease.

For back pain: An acupuncturist will insert from two to 12 needles directly into your back pain area, and sometimes away from your back, in your hand or foot. Once the needles are in, you can often feel your "energy" being stimulated. I often recommend a combination of acupuncture and chiropractic, depending on my diagnosis of the problem. As one of my *Naturally Well* subscribers, you'll discover much more about the application of acupuncture techniques for "what ails you."

✔ Prevent Cataracts Before It's Too Late.

Most people believe—perhaps you included—that cataract formation is part of "normal" aging. Don't believe it. They can be prevented and arrested. You just have to start early enough.

A cataract's main feature is progressive, painless loss of vision as the lens of your eye becomes "cloudy." It's kind of like a transparent egg white turning solid and white in your frying pan. But with the right cataract-prevention savvy, which I write about in *Naturally Well,* you can actually improve and even eliminate early cataract formation without surgery.

Your eye is like the white of an egg

Did you know: The lens of your eye, that tiny little object, has one of the highest concentrations of Vitamin C in your whole body? Taking extra vitamin C regularly is one key weapon to fighting the onset of cataracts. More and more is being learned about cataract prevention, and I'll keep you posted on the approaches that are best for your overall health.

✔ Keep Death From Starting in the Colon.

As dramatic as that sounds, it's a real danger. Waste needs to move along in the intestine without delay. Any unnecessary slowing down increases your likelihood of toxic exposure directly through your intestinal walls and into the blood stream.

Unexpected consequences: Constipation can also be the indirect cause of fatigue, depression, mood swings, lethargy, confusion—and even bad breath. So, for a lot of good reasons, "staying regular" is important for all of us. What it shouldn't be is work. A bowel movement should be a truly satisfying event at least once a day. (I recall hearing a famous actor, being honestly candid about an often taboo subject, describing his two favorite things in life as "a good script and a good BM." We should all have that same attitude.)

The reasons for constipation are many and varied—from thyroid problems to parasites—but often constipation has an emotional and lifestyle component as well. If you have chronic constipation, I'll help you, as a *Naturally Well* subscriber, further explore what you need to do to regain that "smooth move."

Just a F.E.W. solutions to remember: Basic to every effort for more regularity are measures you may already know, but may not know the "why." (F) Eat Fiber (veggies, fruits, grains)—it gives the muscles surrounding your digestive tract something to push against to cause a movement. (E) Exercise—especially walking, running or abdominal routines—this promotes peristalsis

Ways to "take out the trash" everyday

the contractions along the walls of the colon that force the contents forward. W) Water—drinking 6 to 8 glasses a day helps create stool that move more readily.

✔ Beat Back an Illness with Its Own Bat

That is the essence of a very effective healing system called Homeopathy discovered nearly 200 years ago by Samuel Hahnmann, M.D. He

Learn how "like can cure like"

determined that an illness can often be cured by giving a patient tiny doses of a substance that, if given to a

healthy person, would actually produce symptoms of the illness to be cured.

Relief par excellence: Many homeopathic remedies are taken in the form of tiny pellets dissolved under your tongue. For other purposes, there are gels, lotions and ointments. All are completely natural, work gently, have no known side effects and are available at your local health food emporium and many pharmacies. Plus, they all can work rather quickly—for example there

are homeopathic treatments to curtail coughs
and colds, relieve sprains and bruises and stem
infections within minutes after use.

Simple examples: Arnica is the premier
homeopathic first-aid remedy. Take it internally
right after a sprain, a strain or an episode of stiff,
aching muscles. It can decrease the pain rapidly.
But don't use Arnica externally. For that, or any
cut, scrape or boo-boo in life I love a substance
called *Calendula*—it has wonderful soothing,
antimicrobial and wound-healing properties.
And it provides fast, fast relief.

There are so many truly effective homeopathic treatments to recommend for specific
needs, that I make sure to discuss and prescribe
them for you regularly in *Naturally Well* .

EASY REMINDERS

- Garcinia cambogia is a weight loss breakthrough derived from a curry spice.

- Your feelings of depression may be easily
  remedied through nutritional means.

- Chiropractic manipulation can bring a wave of
  relief and relaxation to back problems.

- Acupuncture is an ancient healing art that is
  now considered a modern miracle for pain.

- Cataracts are preventable and reversible—you just have to start early enough.

- Constipation can have emotional and lifestyle causes—and cures.

- Homeopathy offers natural, instantaneous remedies for many of life's bumps, bruises and boo-boos.

CHAPTER 14

Outlive Your Doctor, Your Pharmacist and The Rest of the Medical Establishment.

I said it earlier and I'll say it again here at the end...you can do more to assure your good health and longevity than anyone—including your doctor. And, yes, that means taking aim at your natural biological life expectancy of 120.

Here's the way to do it:

Eat Like a Bushman. There is overwhelming evidence that the healthiest, strongest most disease-resistant cultures ever known were those who lived primarily on whole natural foods. Yet most people have little awareness of how very far we have strayed from the basic diets that human beings evolved with. YOU, on the other hand, are not too late to do something about it. And your body will thank and reward you for it.

Stay Well Like a Medicine Man. Modern medicine, too, has retreated too far from nature, obviously finding the charms of chemistry irre-

112 Outlive Your Doctor

sistible—and more profitable. Instead of developing medicine that supports your body's power to heal itself, (as do Medicine Men of the Rainforest) the emphasis today is on using costly, potent, often-toxic, synthetic drugs. Again, YOU don't have to succumb. And, yes, your body will thank and reward you for it.

Use Your Mind to Reduce Wear and Tear. The state of your mind changes the state of your body. It can heal it or it can tear it down. Your thoughts and feelings always trigger physical reactions of some kind. Can you make sure those reactions are almost always good for your body? Can you make sure your mind is almost always working for good health? Yes—you have that power. And, again, your body will thank and reward you for it.

Begin the journey with a valuable companion: Naturally Well. My monthly Letter is an easy-chair guide to slowing down, and even reversing, the aging process. It is about as far away from a stuffy medical journal as you can get. Instead, it's an eight-page personal letter from me to you. And I want you to know this: Its emphasis is not on getting you to abruptly and jarringly change your life to some idealized state of healthy perfection. No, all *Naturally Well* will do is help you identify the most desirable options you have to stay illness-free and to live longer. And trust me, with natural alternatives, you'll find there are many more kinder, gentler routes to good health than there are harsh, depriving ones.

Please accept these Three Bonuses Just for Giving *Naturally Well* a Look-See.

FREE BONUS #1
Naturally Immune For Life

This Special Report is—without question—a complete education in how to build up your immune system to repel age-related disease. What's more, its easy format enables you to learn a lot in just a little time. You'll quickly discover the 50 most important immunity boosters that promote health and longevity. Plus you'll get the "down side," too—31 everyday immune-depressing things to avoid to prevent premature aging. This unique reference guide also includes my complete directory of natural home remedies, including the most effective phytochemical, vitamin and mineral therapies to reverse the signs of aging and exactly how to use each one. In addition, *Naturally Immune for Life* explains all the ways you can turn your mind into a powerful healer, using techniques that reverse negative emotions and turn them into health-giving attitudes that positively effect every part of your body.

FREE BONUS #2
250 Mouth-Watering Food Remedies
for What Ails You

What great-tasting foods also happen to be
the best medicine for your body? How can you
cure a whole range of typically nagging health
problems just by sitting down and eating foods
you love? The answers to these questions and
many more are in this Special Report—written
for everyone who'd just as well die early if they
had to endure eating boring, tasteless "rabbit
food" to have all the benefits of a healthy
lifestyle. Discover not just one or two, but often
a dozen or more delicious, nourishing food
options for treating everything from arthritis to
skin disorders to intestinal problems to high
blood pressure to depression What foods can
you eat that virtually guarantee a renewed energy you haven't felt in years? How can you eat all
the "gassy" foods you want and not suffer a
moment's discomfort? What natural food flavors—salty, sweet, pungent or sour—should you
emphasize for specific health problems? All
these critical questions and more are yours in
this indispensable volume.

These two extremely important reports are
yours free—and are sent to you immediately
upon indicating that you would like to try a 12-
month subscription to *Naturally Well*.

Subscribe for a risk-free 24 months and receive, in addition, *Cures From the Rainforest Pharmacy*.

Here's an opportunity to benefit *in advance* from the miracle medicines of the coming next century. You'll learn all about them—and how to get them—in my very Special Report on the botanical pharmacy that is the Rainforest. I wrote this report for one reason: There has been precious little investigation by modern medicine into the life-enhancing and life-extending herbs used for so long by tribal peoples. It is now critical for us to take the healing wisdom from thousands of years of experience of medicine men and put it to use protecting our bodies and extending our lives. Learn about such anti-aging substances as *Suma,* considered an effective treatment for many chronic diseases including leukemia, arthritis, asthma, high blood pressure, mononucleosis, candida, hypoglycemia, Epstein-Barr Syndrome, high cholesterol and early stages of cancer. And about *Pau D'Arco,* a powerful anti-bacterial, anti-viral, anti-fungal substance also used to treat ulcers, rheumatism, poor circulation and arthritis. About the bark of the *Jatoba* tree, for renewed energy and about the *Jurubera* plant for improved digestion. Discover page after page of little-known natural remedies that you can benefit from right now.

This important Report is yours in addition to
Naturally Immune for Life and *250 Mouth-
Watering Food Remedies for What Ails You* when
you subscribe for 24 months.

**EXTRA BONUS (while supplies last)
A Special "Try-Me" kit of Remarkable
Natural Home Remedies**

Before you decide to take my advice and
acquire any of the natural remedies I've recommended in this book, wouldn't it be helpful if
you could sample a few first just to experience
their wonderful effects?

Naturally, no store would ever let you do
that, but as a new subscriber to *Naturally Well*,
you'll receive these samples.

By special arrangement with herbal distribu-
tors I know and work with, you will be sent certificates enabling you to receive all of the following, with my compliments.

1 *A Sample of Siberian Ginseng*. This herb is
among the most powerful of the so-called
adaptogens, a class of natural substances known
for their ability to help you dissolve mental and
physical stress. However, the Siberian variety is
extra special in that it also—

• Increases mental alertness and work output.

- Improves work quality under stressful situations, as well as athletic performance.

- Improves your eyesight, hearing and sense of balance.

- Quenches free radicals.

- Boosts your elimination of toxic and harmful waste products and promotes longevity.

- Siberian ginseng makes its benefits known rather quickly.

2 *A Sample of Uña de Gato* This herb is described in independent research as "the most important in the Amazonian Rainforest." That's saying a lot when you consider that more than 200,000 species of plant life have been identified in this vast botanical pharmacy. Uña de Gato is a powerful infection fighter and immune booster. It is used routinely to treat ulcers, skin disorders, gastric disorders, Crohn's disease, genital herpes, colitis, hemorrhoids— all, of course, with zero side effects. It is also considered very effective as a plaque inhibitor, reducing your risk of strokes and heart attacks by inhibiting the formation of plaque in your arteries. There is also evidence that it is responsible for remission of certain cancers and that it provides benefits to arthritis and diabetes patients as well.

3 *A Sample of Marapauma (available in a potent formula called "Warrior").* As I've described, extremely-credible research as well as individuals I spoke with on my trip to the Amazonian Rainforest, indicate that this aphro-disiac (derived from a Brazilian shrub) may pro-vide better results than better-known Yohimbe—and without any side effects. In a study by a renowned French researcher, 262 patients expressing a lack of sexual desire or "erection failures" were given a daily dose of 1 to 1.5 grams of Marapauma.

Within two weeks, 62% of those claiming a loss of libido said that treatment definitely had a positive effect. Fifty-two percent of those with erection problems also felt that Marapauma had helped them.

4 *A Sample of HCA (hydroxycitric acid).* This is a true breakthrough weight loss substance derived from an Asian fruit, Garcinia cambogia. Brandeis University researchers discovered that an extract of Garcina, hydroxycitric acid (HCA), can be a godsend to the overweight individual. It's non-addictive, non-toxic, non-stimulative and its unique chemistry effectively reduces your appetite, and thus your food intake. Even better, it actually stems fat production from the foods you do eat! And while it's doing all that, it also increases your energy level. Finally, and importantly, there is no weight rebound effect after you stop taking it!

100% Protection: My Guarantee of Your Satisfaction.

If you say "yes" to this opportunity to try *Naturally Well,* you'd probably feel more comfortable if it meant "Yes, I'd like to subscribe if I like it after seeing it."

So let's structure it that way. Let me send you a complimentary copy of both my Special Reports, *Naturally Immune for Life* and *250 Mouth-Watering Food Remedies for What Ails You* when you subscribe to *Naturally Well.*

And, if you choose two years of benefit, you can, in addition, discover many miraculous new remedies in *Cures From The Rainforest Pharmacy,* my latest Special Report.

Plus you receive all the Free samples I've described, no matter which subscription you choose.

Then here's my guarantee to you: If you don't start benefiting from the moment you receive your first issue of *Naturally Well,* cancel your subscription anytime within 90 days and I'll see that you receive a 100% refund.

Whatever you decide, all the bonuses are yours to keep with my compliments—even the free samples. They're my way of saying thanks for giving me a try!

■ ■ ■

Thank you for taking the time to read my book. I hope it enlightened you, surprised you, but even more important, motivated you. Because what could be a more worthwhile goal than to *live to age 120 in robust good health?*

Marcus Laux

No-Risk Introductory Subscription Offer

☐ YES, Dr. Laux: I'll accept your offer of the two free bonus reports *Naturally Immune for Life*, and *250 Mouth-Watering Food Remedies for What Ails You* when I begin my trial 12-month subscription to your *Naturally Well* monthly letter for just C$79.95 (a C$20 savings off the regular price). I understand my subscription comes with a 90-day full money back guarantee.

Best Value

☐ I prefer a 24-month subscription to *Naturally Well* for just C$129.95 (I save C$30!) and to receive, in addition, Dr. Laux's Exclusive Report, *Cures from the Rainforest Pharmacy*. This unique publication is mine along with the two Special Reports of one-year subscribers.

Choose your method of payment

☐ Enclosed is my check or money order, payable to *Naturally Well*.
(Please add 7% GST)

☐ Please charge my:

☐ Visa ☐ MasterCard ☐ Discover

Card # _____ Expires _____

Signature _____

Name _____

Address _____

City/State/Zip _____

For Faster Ordering Call Toll-Free 1-800-777-5005

Or send this form to: *Naturally Well*, Phillips Publishing Inc., 1031 Helena St., Fort Erie, Ontario L2A 5N8

GNK400

No-Risk Introductory Subscription Offer

☐ YES, Dr. Laux: I'll accept your offer of the two free bonus reports *Naturally Immune for Life*, and *250 Mouth-Watering Food Remedies for What Ails You* when I begin my trial 12-month subscription to your *Naturally Well* monthly letter for just C$79.95 (a C$20 savings off the regular price). I understand my subscription comes with a 90-day full money back guarantee.

Best Value

☐ I prefer a 24-month subscription to *Naturally Well* for just C$129.95 (I save C$30!) and to receive, in addition, Dr. Laux's Exclusive Report, *Cures from the Rainforest Pharmacy*. This unique publication is mine along with the two Special Reports of one-year subscribers.

Choose your method of payment

☐ Enclosed is my check or money order, payable to *Naturally Well*.

(Please add 7% GST)

☐ Please charge my:

    ☐ Visa ☐ MasterCard ☐ Discover

Name _____

Address _____

Card # _____ Expires _____

City/State/Zip _____

Signature _____

For Faster Ordering Call Toll-Free 1-800-777-5005

Or send this form to: *Naturally Well*, Phillips Publishing Inc., 1031 Helena St., Fort Erie, Ontario L2A 5N8

GNK410

IMPORTANT BONUS

(ONLY while supplies last): Every new subscriber receives certificates for a unique "Try-Me" Kit of Dr. Laux's recommended natural home remedies. You'll just send in your certificates to experience these wonderful cures, with his compliments!

(See back for details)

9

No-Risk Introductory Subscription Offer

☐ YES, Dr. Laux: I'll accept your offer of the two free bonus reports *Naturally Immune for Life*, and *250 Mouth-Watering Food Remedies for What Ails You* when I begin my trial 12-month subscription to your *Naturally Well* monthly letter for just C$79.95 (a C$20 savings off the regular price). I understand my subscription comes with a 90-day full money back guarantee.

Best Value

☐ I prefer a 24-month subscription to *Naturally Well* for just C$129.95 (I save C$30!) and to receive, in addition, Dr. Laux's Exclusive Report, *Cures from the Rainforest Pharmacy*. This unique publication is mine along with the two Special Reports of one-year subscribers.

Choose your method of payment

☐ Enclosed is my check or money order, payable to *Naturally Well*.

(Please add 7% GST)

☐ Please charge my:

    ☐ Visa ☐ MasterCard ☐ Discover

Name _____

Address _____

Card # _____ Expires _____

Signature _____

City/State/Zip _____

For Faster Ordering Call Toll-Free 1-800-777-5005

Or send this form to: *Naturally Well*, Phillips Publishing Inc., 1031 Helena St., Fort Erie, Ontario L2A 5N8

GNK420

IMPORTANT BONUS

(ONLY while supplies last): Every new subscriber receives certificates for a unique "Try-Me" Kit of Dr. Laux's recommended natural home remedies. You'll just send in your certificates to experience these wonderful cures, with his compliments!

(See back for details)

REAP ALL THE BENEFITS OF A TRIAL SUBSCRIPTION TO NATURALLY WELL AT A C$30 SAVINGS—AND RECEIVE TWO BONUS SPECIAL REPORTS.

Naturally Immune for Life is a complete digest on repelling age-related disease. Discover the 50 most important immunity boosters available today, as well as the 31 immunity-depressing influences on your body. Also get a complete directory of natural home remedies, plus proven techniques for reversing the signs of aging. *250 Mouth-Watering Food Remedies for What Ails You* reveals all the tempting foods that just happen to be little-known treatments for many stubborn illnesses. Plus discover the foods that are guaranteed energy boosters, and the specific food flavors—salty, sweet, pungent or sour—you should emphasize for specific health problems.

Additional FREE Report, *Cures from the Rainforest Pharmacy* with your risk-free 24 month subscription.

Dr. Laux's long-anticipated Special Report on the Rainforest is now available and is packed with the best (and often easily obtainable) natural remedies he discovered on his expedition. This exclusive publication is a must! And it's yours along with two other Special Reports *Naturally Immune for Life* and *250 Mouth-Watering Food Remedies for What Ails You* as an honored two-year subscriber.

For Faster Ordering Call Toll-Free 1-800-777-5005

FREE "TRY-ME" KIT OF MIRACLE HOME REMEDIES

As a new subscriber, you receive, with Dr. Laux's compliments, certificates entitling you to a sample of all the following: Siberian Ginseng (amazing stress dissolver), Uña de Gato (#1 immune-enhancing substance from the Rainforest), "Warrior" (contains powerful, proven aphrodisiac), and HCA (a true breakthrough in natural weight loss.)

No-Risk Introductory Subscription Offer

☐ YES, Dr. Laux: I'll accept your offer of the two free bonus reports *Naturally Immune for Life*, and *250 Mouth-Watering Food Remedies for What Ails You* when I begin my trial 12-month subscription to your *Naturally Well* monthly letter for just C$79.95 (a C$20 savings off the regular price). I understand my subscription comes with a 90-day full money back guarantee.

Best Value

☐ I prefer a 24-month subscription to *Naturally Well* for just C$129.95 (I save C$30!) and to receive, in addition, Dr. Laux's Exclusive Report, *Cures from the Rainforest Pharmacy*. This unique publication is mine along with the two Special Reports of one-year subscribers.

Choose your method of payment

☐ Enclosed is my check or money order, payable to *Naturally Well*.
(*Please add 7% GST*)

☐ Please charge my:

☐ Visa ☐ MasterCard ☐ Discover

Card # _____ Expires _____

Signature _____

Name _____

Address _____

City/State/Zip _____

For Faster Ordering Call Toll-Free 1-800-777-5005

Or send this form to: *Naturally Well*, Phillips Publishing Inc., 1031 Helena St., Fort Erie, Ontario L2A 5N8

GNK430

IMPORTANT BONUS

(ONLY while supplies last): Every new subscriber receives certificates for a unique "Try-Me" Kit of Dr. Laux's recommended natural home remedies. You'll just send in your certificates to experience these wonderful cures, with his compliments!

(See back for details)

REAP ALL THE BENEFITS OF A TRIAL SUBSCRIPTION TO NATURALLY WELL AT A C$30 SAVINGS—AND RECEIVE TWO BONUS SPECIAL REPORTS.

Naturally Immune for Life is a complete digest on repelling age-related disease. Discover the 50 most important immunity boosters available today, as well as the 31 immunity-depressing influences on your body. Also get a complete directory of natural home remedies, plus proven techniques for reversing the signs of aging. *250 Mouth-Watering Food Remedies for What Ails You* reveals all the tempting foods that just happen to be little-known treatments for many stubborn illnesses. Plus discover the foods that are guaranteed energy boosters, and the specific food flavors—salty, sweet, pungent or sour—you should emphasize for specific health problems.

Additional FREE Report, *Cures from the Rainforest Pharmacy* with your risk-free 24 month subscription.

Dr. Laux's long-anticipated Special Report on the Rainforest is now available and is packed with the best (and often easily obtainable) natural remedies he discovered on his expedition. This exclusive publication is a must! And it's yours along with two other Special Reports *Naturally Immune for Life* and *250 Mouth-Watering Food Remedies for What Ails You* as an honored two-year subscriber.

For Faster Ordering Call Toll-Free 1-800-777-5005

Or send this form to: *Naturally Well*, Phillips Publishing Inc., 1031 Helena St., Fort Erie,